1

With the aim of reducing the burden of drug expenditures for the elderly, Congress passed the Medicare Modernization Act of 2003, which introduced Medicare Part D in January 2006. The reform led to a substantial expansion in prescription drug insurance coverage. Part D now covers 39 million individuals, and has cost the U.S. government a cumulative \$353 billion.[1] At the time of its inception, Medicare Part D represented the largest expansion of an entitlement program since the implementation of Medicare. Despite the enormous size of the program, there exists little evidence of any benefits of Medicare Part D in terms of health outcomes.

This study presents new evidence on the impact of Medicare Part D, and more broadly, the effect of prescription drug coverage expansion on mortality. There are several reasons to believe that the reform may have had an impact on mortality. Nearly half of drug expenditures are spent on treatments to prevent cardiovascular-related deaths. These drugs include some of the most innovative and effective treatments for preventing heart disease, the leading cause of death in the United States. Second, the Act improved the affordability of prescription drugs. The financial incentives from expanding drug insurance may be particularly important, since before the reform prescription drugs accounted for around 42 percent of out-of-pocket spending, even though drugs accounted for just 18 percent of total medical expenditures. In addition, numerous studies have shown that financial incentives encourage the chronically ill to start treatment and also improve adherence to medications (Eaddy et al. (2012), Solomon et al.(2009) and Cutler and Everett (2010)).

By contrast, Medicare Part D may have had only a limited effect on mortality, if, for instance, those individuals in need of prescription drugs had already purchased prescription drug insurance before the reform. That is, the impact on mortality of prescription drug coverage expansion is likely to be less than under random assignment. Overall, it remains unclear whether Medicare Part D had any impact on the mortality rate of elder individuals.

Our identification strategy relies on geographic differences in insurance coverage across U.S. counties before the reform's implementation. Using the Medicare Current Beneficiary Survey (MCBS), we estimate demographically adjusted rates of prescription drug coverage for age 65+ Medicare enrollees across counties before the implementation of Part D. We find that those areas with lower levels of coverage before the reform experienced greater drug insurance expansion as a result of Part D.[2] This information is combined with county-

---

[1]Source: Congressional Budget Office, 2014.

[2]We also show that pre-reform levels of drug insurance are strongly and negatively related to the observed increase in drug coverage post-reform, providing the basis for the identification strategy applied in this paper.

level mortality data obtained from the Centers for Disease Control and Prevention (CDC) for the years 2000 to 2010.

While this type of geographic variation has been employed in other studies,[3] there are two additional factors introduced in this study that are critical for identifying the effects on mortality. First, it is important to analyze the effects of mortality by disease category. Specifically, we find strong persistence in the disease-specific cause of death within counties over time, so county-disease fixed effects are important for accounting for the health across these populations. Indeed, we find that assessing mortality by disease leads to a more accurate measure of the effects on mortality.

Second, it is essential to consider how the reform affects the population's health in future periods. If drug insurance expansion is successful it will improve the survival of individuals on the margin of dying—that is, those that have relatively poor health. This implies that in subsequent periods the population of individuals living with a serious chronic health condition will increase. Considering this type of dynamic effect, which we call "delayed mortality," is crucial when studying health care and mortality in the United States since chronic conditions account for 75 percent of health care costs and cause seven out of ten deaths each year.[4] For this reason, it is important to measure the effects of the reform on mortality when the health of the population affected by the reform is most similar to the pre-reform population, which is precisely when the reform takes effect. To account for effects of the reform in subsequent periods, we find that it is critical to incorporate the likely change in the population's health caused by the reform.

We focus on measuring the effects of mortality on two categories: (1) cardiovascular-related conditions (e.g., heart disease, stroke, and heart attacks) and (2) all other conditions (e.g., cancers and pneumonia). To measure the effects of the reform on mortality, our main results focus on a relatively short time period around the reform. Specifically, we measure one year mortality rates at three points in time: July 1, 2003, to June 30, 2004; July 1, 2004, to June 30, 2005; and July 1, 2006, to June 30, 2007.[5] Importantly, this study focuses on those individuals dying between July 1, 2006, and June 30, 2007, since this is the

---

[3]This approach is similar to Finkelstein (2007) looking at the effects of the 1965 introduction of Medicare and Dunn and Shapiro (2015) looking at the effects of Massachusetts insurance reform.

[4]These statistics are from the Centers of Disease Control and Prevention (http://www.cdc.gov/chronicdisease/overview/).

[5]The results using June 2005 to June 2006 produce similar results, although it is potentially contaminated for a couple of reasons. First, it may include consumers who change purchasing patterns in anticipation of the reform. Second, it includes a mix of individuals before 2006 that are unaffected by the reform and those after 2006 that may be affected.

population that is initially affected by the reform.[6] Using this time period we find that the probability of a cardiovascular-related mortality drops significantly, while mortality rates for noncardiovascular causes of death remain statistically unchanged. Estimates suggest that between 19,000 and 27,000 more individuals were alive in mid-2007 because of the Part D implementation in mid-2006.

We conduct numerous robustness checks to confirm the reduction in cardiovascular-related mortality is statistically significant. For example, using the full pre-reform period from 2000-04 and including county-specific or county-disease-specific trends produces similar results. As an additional check on our identification strategy, we apply a triple-difference analysis that combines mortality data from both the 65+ and 55-64 populations, and we find that cardiovascular-related deaths for the 65+ decline significantly more due to the reform relative to the under-65 population in the same county. Additional extensions of the basic model demonstrate the importance of accounting for the changing health of the population caused by the reform. Specifically, after controlling for Part D's effect on the population's health, we find that the reform significantly lowers cardiovascular-related deaths over the entire 2006-10 period.

To better understand the total value of the Part D expansion, we measure the effects of Part D on prescription drug expenditures using the MCBS data. As would be expected, those areas predicted to be most affected by the reform had the largest increase in drug expenditures. Overall, the reforms are associated with a 30 percent reduction in out-of-pocket cost sharing and a 10 percent increase in drug expenditures. We find that the predicted changes in the response to the reform imply a price elasticity of demand of -0.26, which corresponds roughly to the estimates found in the RAND study (Newhouse (1993) and other more recent evidence based on a natural experiment for the Medicare population (e.g., Chandra et al. (2010)).[7]

The growth in expenditures caused by the reform are compared to the monetized benefit of lives saved with the aim to better understand the overall value of the reform. Based on a $200,000 monetary value of a life-year,[8] we find that the additional value of life-years gained is between $3.9 and $5.4 billion, which greatly exceeds the additional out-of-pocket costs for cardiovascular-related drugs of approximately $870 million. In fact, the total

---

[6]Ketcham and Simon (2008) use large monthly pharmaceutical data that highlight the timing of Part D effects. It appears most of the impact on out-of-pocket cost and utilization occurred by early to mid-2006.

[7]Using the predicted change in drug insurance coverage as an instrumental variable, we also provide a more direct estimate of a demand elasticity using individual-level data with estimates that range from -0.17 to -0.26.

[8]This is the amount applied in Eggleston et al. (2011).

benefit exceeds the total estimated additional spending on cardiovascular drugs from the program of \$3.8 billion. Even lower estimates of the additional value of life-years gained are around \$1.9 to \$2.7 billion, still exceeding the additional out-of-pocket cost. When the financial risk protection of the program is also considered (see Engelhardt and Gruber (2011)) it is likely that the benefits of the program greatly outweighed the deadweight loss of the reform across all scenarios.[9]

Although this study assesses solely prescription drug expansion, it is related to a broader literature discussing the link between health insurance and health outcomes. The well-known RAND study, a randomized trial of health insurance coverage across the population (Newhouse (1993)), found that insurance generosity had only a limited impact on health. More recently, a randomized experiment in Oregon found no statistically significant relationship between Medicaid coverage and measured physical outcomes after two years (Baicker et al. (2013)). By contrast, Card, Dobkin and Maestas (2009) apply regression discontinuity analysis and find lower mortality rates and higher service utilization for Medicare patients admitted to emergency departments, relative to individuals under age 65.[10] Our study shows that a subset of health insurance, specifically prescription drug coverage, has had clear positive effects on health outcomes, mainly stemming from the improved health for those with cardiovascular-related diseases. It is important to emphasize that this paper measures the estimated lives saved by the Part D program due to insurance expansion. Prior to the expansion, one may expect that those with the highest need for prescription drugs would have purchased insurance, if possible. For this reason, we expect the expansion effect to understate the full effect on mortality relative to randomized assignment.

1   Background on Medicare Part D and Drug Spending

Medicare was established in 1965 and provides insurance coverage to those age 65 and older, as well as certain disabled populations. Although the program covered most medical care expenditures, such as hospital and doctor office expenditures, it did not cover

---

[9]Engelhardt and Gruber (2011) measure the value of financial risk protection from the Part D program and find that it roughly equals the deadweight loss of financing Part D. Their cost-benefit analysis did not consider the potential health benefits of the Part D program.

[10]An examination of the introduction of Medicare in 1965 shows no effect of Medicare expansion on mortality (Finkelstein and McKnight (2008).

prescription drug costs. In 1965 this was not viewed as a serious omission, since prescription drugs accounted for only a small fraction of total expenditures. However, in subsequent years numerous breakthroughs in the pharmaceutical sector led to innovative treatments that greatly increased expenditures on prescription drugs. Just before the reform, the total average per capita expenditures on prescription drugs for the 65+ population was $1,743 per year in 2004-05 (about 18 percent of total medical expenditures).

With the aim of reducing the burden of drug expenditures for the elderly, Congress passed the Medicare Modernization Act of 2003, which introduced Medicare Part D in January 2006 and led to a substantial expansion in prescription drug coverage. Unlike traditional fee-for-service Medicare that is administered by the federal government, Medicare Part D coverage is offered through private-sector insurers that are under contract with the government. Individuals can obtain insurance through three distinct alternatives. One option is to purchase a stand-alone Medicare Prescription Drug Plan (PDP), that offers prescription-drug benefits. Another option is to purchase a private Medicare Advantage plan, an alternative to traditional fee-for-service Medicare, that provides all the benefits associated with fee-for-service Medicare but often includes additional benefits, such as prescription drug coverage. The third option is to retain their existing drug coverage that they received through their current employer, as long as the plan's benefits are comparable to the generosity of a standard Part D plan or better.[11]

Indeed, the passage of Medicare Part D had a large effect on the number of people with drug insurance coverage. Using measures constructed in this paper, in 2004 around 67 percent of the elderly Medicare population had drug coverage, but that percentage grew to more than 90 percent by 2007. However, connecting the measure of drug insurance expansion to changes in mortality rates is challenging, as illustrated in Figure 1. Figure 1 shows the trend in mortality rates for the 65+ population for both cardiovascular and noncardiovascular causes, along with the fraction of the population with drug insurance. The graph illustrates two points. First, there appears to be no obvious effect of drug insurance coverage on either category of mortality at the national level.[12] Second, the mortality rate for cardiovascular-related conditions is falling over the entire time period, suggesting the increased use of prescription drugs to treat cardiovascular-related conditions

---

[11]In 2006, a standard Part D plan included no coverage for the first $250 in drug costs for each year. The plan covered 75 percent of the cost for the next $2,250, 0 percent of the drug expenditures for the next $3,600, and 95 percent of drug spending above $5,100.

[12]About 1.8 million individuals over the age of 65 die each year, so it may be challenging to identify the thousands of individuals who lived due to Part D reform using national aggregate mortality statistics.

is likely a contributing factor to this decline.[13]

Figure 1: Mortality and Drug Coverage Over the Reform Period

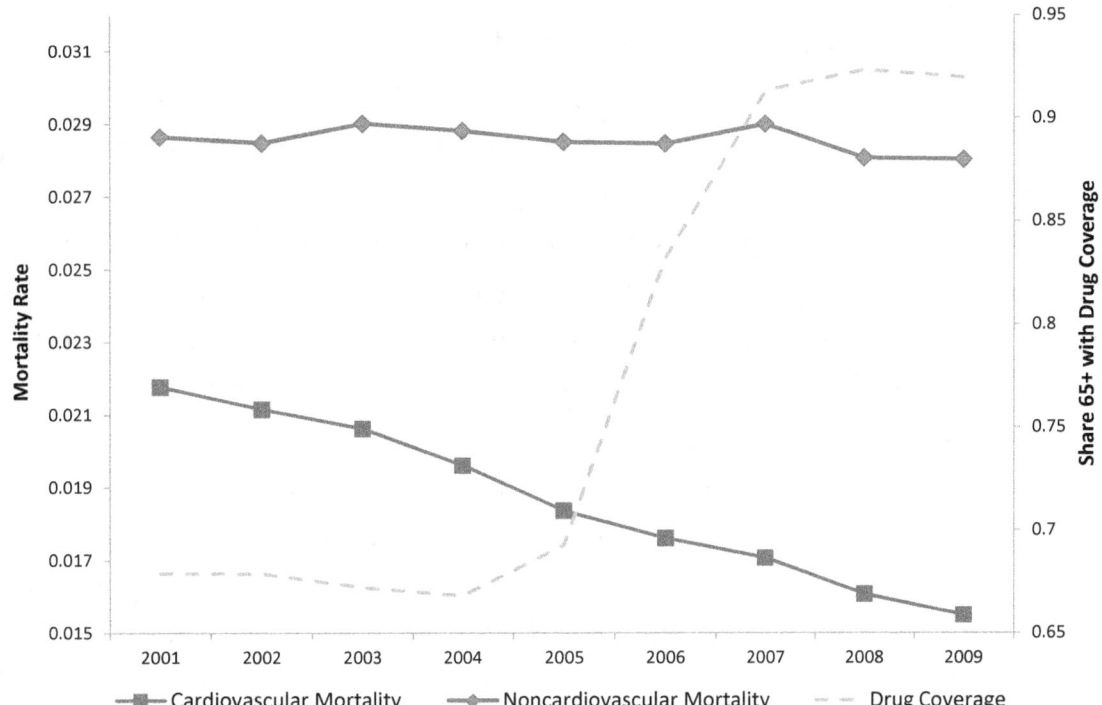

Notes: Authors' calculations based on CDC and MCBS data.

The MCBS dataset used to estimate drug coverage in Figure 1 is not large enough to investigate the precise timing (i.e., month) that Part D had an effect on prescription drug utilization, since some purchases of Part D plans occurred later in 2006. However, work by Ketcham and Simon (2008), which uses a large database of pharmacy claims, finds that most of the expansion in prescription drug utilization occurred quite rapidly in the first few months of 2006. Therefore, considering mid-2006 to mid-2007 as the initial 12 months that Part D would have an impact on mortality seems appropriate.

While the trend of falling cardiovascular-related deaths occurred both before and after the reform, this entire period is also marked by a continued rise in the use of cardio-vascular drugs. Figure 2 divides cardiovascular-related drug use into the number of pre-scription drug purchases for the 65+ population by drug category, with the bottom three

---

[13]Cutler (2004) argues that roughly one-third of the decline in cardiovascular-related mortality may be attributable to innovative prescription drugs that control hypertension and high cholesterol. The growth in anticholesterol drug use is particularly rapid in the early 2000s (see Dunn (2012)).

shades accounting for the major cardiovascular drug categories. These three therapeutic classes of drugs are particularly effective at treating cardiovascular illnesses and preventing cardiovascular-related deaths. The largest category is antihyperlipidemic agents, which is a category of drugs used to treat high cholesterol, one of the leading causes of heart disease. In numerous clinical trials, anticholesterol drugs have proven effective at reducing cardiovascular deaths (LaRosa et al. (1999) and Law et al. (2003)) and this category of drugs underwent substantial expansion and innovation in the preceding decade (Dunn (2012)). The second category of cardiovascular agents includes a variety of antihypertensive drugs used to treat high blood pressure, such as oral diuretics, calcium channel blockers, beta-blockers, angiotensin-converting enzyme (ACE) inhibitors, and angiotension-receptor antagonists, all of which have been shown to substantially reduce the risk of mortality, stroke and heart attacks (Cutler et al. (2007)). The smallest of these three categories, based on expenditures, is the coagulation modifiers. Coagulation modifiers include a variety of drugs that are used to prevent clots from forming in blood vessels and to prevent strokes. Like other categories of drugs, these have also been proven highly effective in reducing cardiovascular-related mortalities (Antithrombotic Trialists' Collaboration (2002)). Combined, these three drug categories account for 48 percent of expenditures for individuals 65 and older over the 2003-09 period, and they account for an even greater share of pharmacy purchases, around 53 percent.[14]

Most of these types of cardiovascular drugs have been shown to have an immediate impact on an individual's health. The timing of the benefits of drugs used to treat hypertension is well documented. For instance, two well-known clinical trials performed in the 1960s by the Veterans Administration Cooperate Study Group (VACG (1967, 1970)) found strong evidence that hypertension drugs are effective within a small time frame. One trial consisted of 143 male hypertensive patients with very high diastolic blood pressure, averaging between 115 and 129 mm Hg. Over the course of the trial period, there were no deaths in the treated group and four deaths in the placebo group. Three of these four deaths occurred within the first six months of the trial period. The second VACG trial examined hypertensive males with less severe diastolic blood pressure—between 90 and 114 mm Hg. Drug treatment was shown to reduce the risk of death from 55 percent to 18 percent over a five-year period, with effects beginning in the first year of treatment.

More recent clinical trials of drugs used to treat hypertension have been conducted

---

[14]Estimates obtained from Medical Care Expenditure Panel Survey data. The same drug categories were not reported consistently in the years prior to 2003, so only post-2003 prescription drug purchases are shown in Figure 2.

on older patients, as well as patients with isolated systolic hypertension. For instance, a trial by the SHEP Cooperate Research Group (SHEP (1991)) examined the effect of a low-dosage of chlorthalidone on individuals over the age of 60. The trial found that the incidence of total stroke (i.e., fatal and nonfatal) was reduced by 36 percent over five years, with large effects within 18 months of treatment (see Figure 2 of the study on page 3259). Results from the Swedish Trial in Old Patients with Hypertension (Dahlof et al. (1991)), focused on older individuals (ages 70 to 84) with hypertension. The study found that drug treatment reduced the risk of death within one year of treatment.

Results from clinical trials on statins began being reported in the early 1990s. The Cholesterol Treatment Trialists' (CTT) Collaboration summed up many of these trials in a meta-analysis based on individual patient data. The study showed efficacy across a broad range of patients (CTT Collaborators (2005)). In particular, there was a large reduction in fatal coronary heart disease and nonfatal myocardial infarction in the first year of treatment. Certain studies show large immediate impacts on mortality for sicker individuals. For instance, a study by the Blood Pressure Lowering Treatment Trialists' Collaboration (BPLTT Collaboration 2003) examined the impact of atorvastatin on patients with lower-than-average cholesterol, but who had hypertension. The study showed that the risk of fatal coronary heart disease or non-fatal myocardial infarction fell significantly in the first year of follow-up. A later meta-analysis by the CTT (CTT Collaborators 2008) showed similarly strong effects on mortality for patients with and without diabetes within one year of treatment. More recent meta-analyses have shown that statins may reduce major cardiovascular events for patients without any cardiovascular disease (CTT Collaborators 2010, 2012).

From Figure 1 we do not observe any sharp changes in mortality rates, despite the substantial evidence that Part D increased prescription drug utilization (i.e., Lichtenberg and Sun (2007), Ketcham and Simon (2008), Khan and Kaestner (2009), and Duggan and Scott-Morton (2010)). To identify the effects of Part D on mortality, this paper exploits geographic differences in drug insurance coverage before the reform. Prior to the reform, drug insurance coverage across geographic markets was influenced by several factors, such as the availability of Medicare Advantage plans, which frequently offered drug coverage. Drug coverage was also influenced by the eligibility requirements for Medicaid in the state, and the prevalence of employers offering prescription drug coverage to retirees. As we show later, those areas that had lower levels of drug coverage before the reform are also the areas that had higher levels of expansion.

An alternative strategy for identifying the effects of reform on mortality is to see how

Figure 2: Prescription Drug Purchases Over the Reform Period

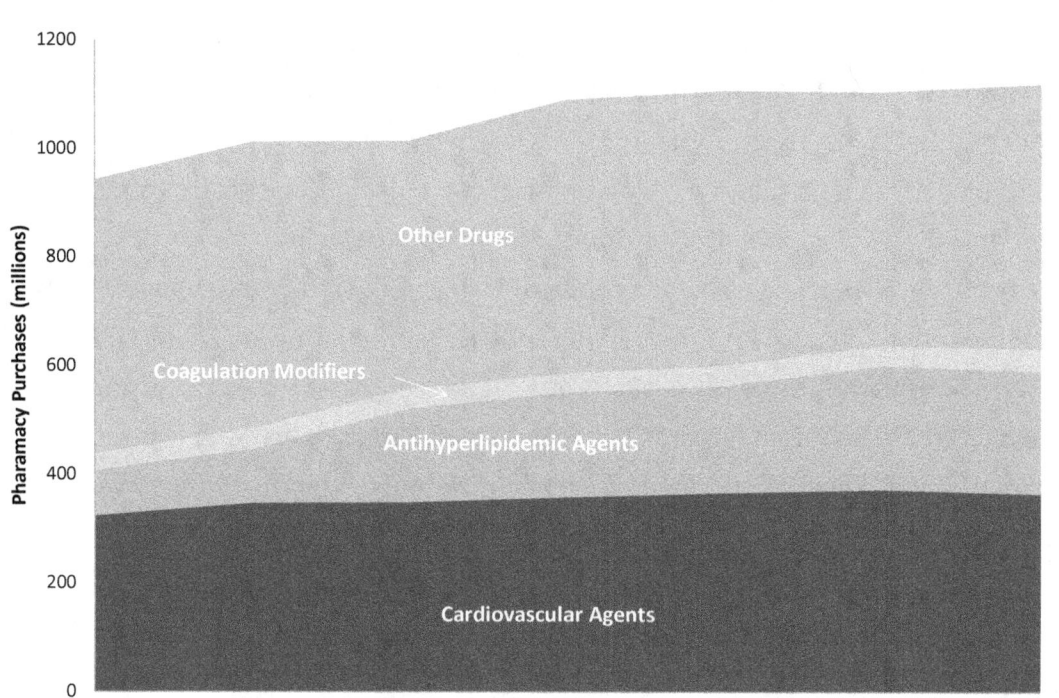

Notes: Authors' calculations based on data from the Medical Expenditure Panel Survey.

mortality rates of individuals aged 65 and over have changed relative to a younger but comparable population, the population aged 55-64. Indeed, we also exploit this difference to conduct falsification exercises. However, a major issue with this approach is that around 7 percent of the 55-64 population ages qualify for Medicare based on their disabilities, but this insurance information is not available in the mortality data. This population is relatively unhealthy, accounting for around 18 percent of total medical expenditures for the 55-64 age category, and the reported rate of cardiovascular conditions in this population is actually much more prevalent than in the 65-69 age range.[15] Therefore, the introduction of Part D will likely have a disproportionate effect on the mortality of the Medicare subpopulation in the 55-64 age range, potentially leading to an underestimation of the total

[15]For instance, 11 percent of the 55-64 population have atherosclerosis, while just 7 percent of the 65-69 population have this condition. Hypertension and diabetes are also more prevalent in the 55-64 Medicare population. This estimate is obtained from the MCBS data for the years 2001-2009. Overall, about 15 percent of Medicare enrollees are under 65.

mortality effect. Moreover, there may be spillover effects, since the increase in the use of prescription drugs by the elderly could lead to increased use for other populations through a number of mechanisms.[16] Although comparing to the under 55-64 population could substantially understate the effects of Part D, we do conduct some comparisons across these populations as additional evidence of identification.

2 Drug Insurance Coverage Expansion and Expected Effects on Mortality

Assessing the impact of drug insurance expansion on mortality is not a straightforward task because it includes a number of empirical challenges. Thus, we begin by discussing the hypothetical effects of an insurance expansion on mortality rates. This discussion highlights the challenges in measuring the effects of insurance on mortality and also helps motivate our empirical approach.

Figure 3 shows a hypothetical effect of drug insurance expansion on mortality. On the X-axis of the figure is a timeline and the Y-axis includes the two main mortality rates studied in this paper, cardiovascular-related mortality and noncardiovascular-related mortality. We normalize the mortality rate for both categories to 4 percent before the the reform. The annual mortality rate is measured over a one-year period and represents the share of the population that dies in the following year, which is calculated based on a ratio of the number of deaths in the following year divided by the total population. For example, the mortality rate in period t captures the share of the population at time $t - 1$ that dies over the following year. The timeline includes the pre-Part D period when mortality rates are constant, as well as the point of drug insurance expansion at time period $t - 1$.

Panel A shows the impact on the mortality rate under the assumption that prescription drugs have a large beneficial health effect on cardiovascular-related illnesses. Here there is a permanent decline in the level of cardiovascular mortality rate, and no impact on the noncardiovascular mortality rate. Panel A, however, ignores the fact that those saved by the reform are likely in poor health status—that is, they are on the margin of dying. This poses two additional likely effects of the Medicare Part D health reform.

First, those individuals saved by the reform likely have numerous comorbidities. Once

---

[16]These could be either social effects of peers, effects through the prescribing patterns of physicians, or the impact of expanding the private insurance market on bargaining for the non-Medicare commercial market (see Lakdawalla and Yin (2014)).

11

saved, these individuals are more likely to die of an alternative cause. In other words, different disease categories are competing risks. Second, those individuals saved by the reform likely have more severe forms of cardiovascular or noncardiovascular disease, and therefore represent a sicker population. Thus, the periods after the reform will appear to have a less healthy population, which increases the proportion of those dying from any disease. Similar types of "harvesting" effects have been documented by researchers studying the impact of weather and air quality on mortality (e.g., Lee (1981), Hajat et al. (2002), Schwartz (2001), and Deschenes and Moretti (2009)), but to our knowledge, this phenomenon has not been studied in the context of Medicare Part D.

These two additional effects are included in Panel B. The competing-risks effect causes the mortality rate for noncardiovascular deaths to *increase*—once being saved, the individual is more likely to die of something other then cardiovascular disease.[17] The delayed-mortality effect causes both cardiovascular- and noncardiovascular-related mortality to increase in later periods. This reflects the fact that those (likely sicker) individuals saved from a cardiovascular-related death in period t enter the population of period $t+1$, raising the mortality rate for *any* cause.[18]

The magnitude of these effects will depend on the health of the population that survives due to reform. Interestingly, we should expect that the health of the population in the post-reform periods will be quite distinct from the population in the pre-reform period, precisely when the effect on mortality is larger. Therefore, one might expect this secondary effect to be strongest in those areas where Part D has the greatest impact.

The parameters used in constructing Figure 3 were chosen for illustrative purposes, but the patterns in this figure offer several insights that will help guide the measurement of the effects on mortality. One lesson implied by Figure 3 is that identifying the timing of the effects of the reform is critical. Measuring the effects of reform on mortality in later periods may not accurately capture the effects of the reform. For example, the mortality rate several years after the reform might look similar to the mortality rate before the reform simply because the post-reform population includes sicker individuals previously saved by the reform. Therefore, in order to identify the effects of insurance expansion on

---

[17]This illustrative figure is based on a simulation that posits:

Pr(dying from a noncardio disease in t | "saved" by reform in t) = 20%.

[18]This illustrative figure is based on a simulation that posits:

Pr(dying from any disease in t + 1 | "saved" by reform in t) = 50%

Pr(dying .... t + 2 | "saved" .... t, lives to t + 1) = 25%

Pr(dying .... t + 3 | "saved" .... t, lives to t + 2) = 12.5%

Pr(dying .... t + 4 | "saved" .... t, lives to t + 3) = 6.25%

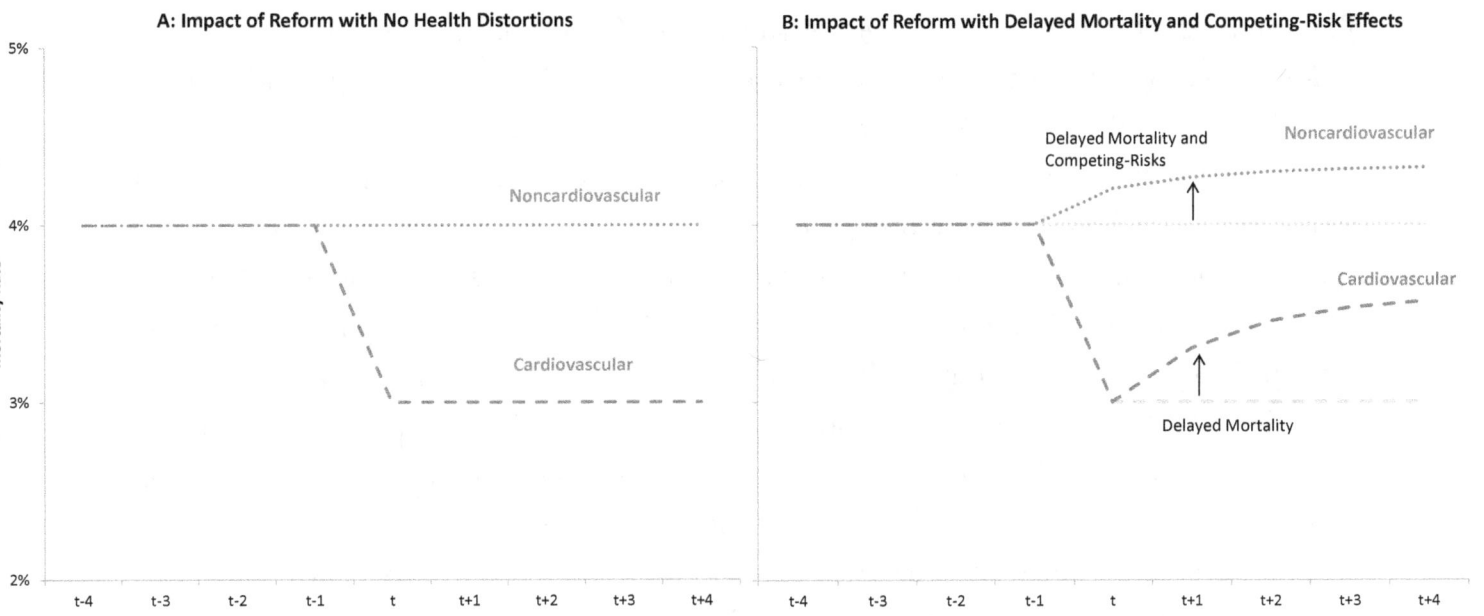

Figure 3: Hypothetical Effects of Drug Insurance Expansion

mortality in later periods, it may be important to account for the changes in the health of the population caused by the reforms. Another lesson learned from Figure 3 is that the changes in the disease-specific mortality rates are more stark and easily identified in the data, relative to total mortality. Specifically, competing risks may cause the time-series pattern of the disease-specific mortality rates to move in distinct directions from the overall mortality rate, which is useful for identifying the effects of the reform.

3   Data

The data for this study are from two main sources. One data source is the MCBS data from 2000 to 2009. The MCBS is an annual survey administered by the Center for Medicare and Medicaid Services (CMS) that randomly surveys about 12,000 individuals from the full Medicare population each year. The second data source is the micro mortality data from the Centers for Disease Control and Prevention (CDC). These two data sources are described below. Additional data sources are also incorporated in our analysis and will be discussed briefly at the end of this section.

The MCBS data contain a variety of demographic and medical-care information on individuals in the survey. The demographics include the age, sex, education, income, and perceived health status of the individuals. The survey also includes questions regarding 26 specific health conditions. In addition to these questions, the survey also covers information about individual insurance enrollment. Although all individuals in the sample are covered by Medicare, the generosity of the drug insurance coverage may vary greatly. For instance, an individual could have a Medicaid plan, a Medicare Advantage plan, or a variety of supplemental insurance plans, such as Medigap or retiree drug coverage. Within each plan category, the level of generosity can also vary by a large amount and the available options often changed as a result of the introduction of Part D. For instance, after the introduction of Part D, those individuals who received their prescription drug coverage through Medicaid were automatically enrolled in Part D. The MCBS data also include expenditure information, including total expenditures for all services as well as out-of-pocket expenditures. Expenditure information is also provided by category, including prescription drug expenditures and out-of-pocket drug expenditures.

Table 1 provides some basic descriptive statistics on the Medicare population over the age of 65 around the time of implementation from 2004-07. The first point to note is that a substantial fraction of the 65+ Medicare population has cardiovascular-related conditions. Around 20 percent of the sample has a serious heart-related condition (including arteriosclerotic heart disease, heart attack, angina, congestive heart failure, or other heart conditions) that likely puts them at a high risk of cardiovascular death. In addition, 49 percent report having hypertension and 22 percent have diabetes, which are key risk factors for developing more serious heart conditions. Another feature of this older demographic is that they tend to be afflicted by other serious health conditions. For example, around 9 percent of the population is reported to have some type of cancer. For this older population, these various conditions should be viewed as competing risks that often appear together. For instance, two-thirds of individuals reporting cancer also report having diabetes, hypertension, or some severe heart condition.[19]

The bottom of Table 1 reports some summary information on the observed expenditures in this data both before and after the reform. A particularly noticeable difference pre- and post- reform is the large change in the share of expenditures that is paid out-of-pocket, falling from 31.1 percent prior to the reform to 23.3 percent. Therefore, as expected, Part D appears to cause an increase in the generosity of drug benefits, but the share of spending

---

[19]This health information does not represent the actual health of the population, since it is determined by the responses of the survey participants, who may be unaware of health conditions. For instance, until individuals have a cholesterol test they may be unaware of having high cholesterol.

for nonprescription drug services paid out-of-pocket barely changes.

Table 1: Descriptive Statistics for Age 65+ Population

Variable	mean	90th pctl.	10th pctl.
Health and Demographics			
Age	75.83	66	87
Male	0.42		
Household Income	$33,937	$8,652	$60,000
College (Bachelor Degree)	0.17		
BMI	26.90	20.98	33.47
Health			
Serious Heart Condition	0.20		
Hypertension	0.49		
Diabetes	0.22		
Cancer	0.09		
Cancer and Other Heart-Related Condition	0.06		
Expenditures			
Pre-Reform (2004-2005)			
Average Total Expenditures Drugs	$1,743		
Average Out-of-pocket Expenditures Drugs	$543		
Share of Expenditures Out-of-Pocket - Drugs	31.1%		
Average Total Expenditures (Excluding Drugs)	$7,873		
Average Out-of-pocket Expenditures (Excluding Drugs)	$726		
Share of Expenditures Out-of-Pocket (Excluding Drugs)	9.2%		
Post-Reform (2006-2007)			
Average Total Expenditures Drugs	$2,196		
Average Out-of-pocket Expenditures Drugs	$512		
Share of Expenditures Out-of-Pocket - Drugs	23.3%		
Average Total Expenditures (Excluding Drugs)	$8,710		
Average Out-of-pocket Expenditures (Excluding Drugs)	$875		
Share of Expenditures Out-of-Pocket (Excluding Drugs)	10.0%		

In this paper, whether an individual has drug coverage or not is defined using a combination of survey information from the individual that indicates drug insurance coverage, and expenditure information. The survey information from individuals includes whether they have drug insurance through Medicaid, Medicare Advantage (the private component of Medicare), or an alternative supplementary drug plan. Benefit structures can vary widely across plans and may also change before and after implementation as the competitive landscape and offerings shift. For this reason, we refine our prescription drug insurance indicator by incorporating reported out-of-pocket and total prescription drug expenditure information into our definition of drug coverage to ensure that the expenditure information does not contradict the coverage variable from the survey.[20]

---

[20]Specifically, for those individuals who have more than $100 in total drug expenditures, we indicate

The MCBS data are used in two aspects of this paper. First, the MCBS data are used to estimate both the pre-reform drug insurance coverage across geographic areas, as well as the predicted change in the insurance rate due to the reform. This is essential for identification of the mortality effect of the reform and will be discussed further in the following subsection. Second, the MCBS data are used to examine how the reform impacts prescription drug expenditures.

The second data source is mortality data from the CDC. The mortality data include information on every death in the United States from 2000 to 2010. They include the age, sex, specific cause of death, and the county of the death for each individual in the United States who died over the sample period. The cause of death is listed as a precise diagnosis that we aggregate to more broadly defined disease chapters. In this paper we classify "cardiovascular deaths" as all causes of death that fall under the chapter category called "diseases of the circulatory system" in the International Classification of Diseases, Ninth Revision (ICD-9).[21] These causes of death include atherosclerosis, heart attacks, and various types of heart disease. As discussed previously, the key therapeutic classes mentioned above target the major conditions in this category. Table D1 reports the frequency by disease chapter in the Appendix of this paper, which shows that 40 percent of all deaths are cardiovascular deaths. For simplicity, most of this paper focuses primarily on just two cause-of-death categories, (1) cardiovascular-related deaths and (2) noncardiovascular-related deaths (i.e., all others). After using these categories to demonstrate the main points, later sections will demonstrate some insights from expanding the analysis to incorporate alternative cause-of-death categories. To construct mortality rate estimates for each county, the mortality data are combined with information about the population in each county taken from the intercessional estimates of the U.S. Census Bureau, which is a population estimate for July 1 of each year. The annual mortality rate is computed by dividing the total deaths from July 1 to June 30 of the following year by the total population estimate for July 1 of the initial year. The broad national trends for

---

people as having drug insurance if they pay less than 20 percent of the total expenditures out-of-pocket and we mark them as not having drug coverage if they pay more than 80 percent of expenditures out-of-pocket. Survey information indicating drug insurance status is used for those individuals who have less than $100 in drug expenditures and those individuals who pay less than 80 percent out-of-pocket, but more than 20 percent. We explore alternative drug coverage definitions, but they produce qualitatively similar results.

[21]Specifically, the data provide cause of death by ICD-10 codes. Since ICD-9 codes have been more broadly used in the health literature, we use a disease-crosswalk to map these codes to broadly defined ICD-9 disease chapters (http://www.nber.org/data/icd9-icd-10-cm-and-pcs-crosswalk-general-equivalence-mapping.html).

these two causes of death are shown in Figure 1, discussed previously.[22]

There are two measurements of mortality assessed in this paper. One measurement is a basic ratio of the number of deaths from period t to $t+1$ divided by the population in period t. In these estimates, the mortality rates are constructed by sex and five-year age categories up to the age of 84. The Census also reports total population for males and females age 85 and older, but there are no five-year age categories. Since age adjustment cannot be performed for those individuals 85 and over, our preferred mortality rate measures are for the age 65 to 84 population.[23] An overall mortality rate is constructed by weighting the population in each age-sex bin based on the overall population in that category for the year 2000, so that mortality rates are comparable across counties and over time.[24]

One issue with this mortality measure is that it treats the death of a 65-year-old person and an 84-year-old person equally, even though the total years-of-life-lost (YLL) are likely greater when a 65-year-old individual dies than when an 84-year-old individual dies. To better reflect the total YLL, we construct an alternative measure in which deaths are weighted by the expected years of life lost for each age category.[25] The age- and sex-adjusted YLL is our preferred measure of mortality since it is a more precise measure of life saved. We also focus on the 65 to 84 age range because age adjustment cannot be performed for those dying in the 85+ range, although we report results for all age ranges in the Appendix. To reduce small-sample bias, we include only those counties with at least 2,000 individuals 65 and over, which implies about 30 to 40 cardiovascular deaths per year in the county.[26]

---

[22]We use CDC data rather than Medicare claims data to study the impact of Part D on mortality for two reasons. First, we are not aware of any available sample of claims for the full Medicare Advantage population. Second, even if claims data were available, it may be challenging to use this information to control for the health of the population, since the observation of diseases in the claims will be biased toward those who seek medical care. In contrast, the death certificates are more likely to be uniformly measured across populations and over time.

[23]Results for the overall 65+ population are included in Appendix Table D8.

[24]Let $Share_{00}^{65-69}$ be the share of the population above 65 that is in the age 65-69 age range in 2000. Let $Mort_{d,t}^{65-69}$ be the mortality rate in the 65-69 age range with disease d at time t to $t+1$. Then the overall mortality rate is constructed as a weighted average of the population share: $\sum_{a \in \{65-69,...,80-84, and 85+\}} Mort_{d,t}^a \cdot Share_{00}^a$.

[25]Specifically, we use data on the Actuarial Life tables from the Social Security website (http://www.ssa.gov/OACT/STATS/table4c6.html). Let the life expectancy for individuals in age range, a, be denoted, L^a. The mortality rate that values the years of potential life lost is calculated as: $\sum_{a \in \{65-69,...,80-84, and 85+\}} Mort_{d,t}^a \cdot Share_{00}^a \cdot L^a$.

[26]See Appendix Table D5 for a list of those counties used in our analysis. We report results with no population cut-off in Appendix Table D8.

In addition to the above data, our analysis also incorporates annual unemployment data at the county level from the Bureau of Labor Statistics. While much of the analysis in this paper looks over a relatively short time period and uses county-disease fixed effects that lessen the need for detailed controls for population health, the unemployment rate has been shown to be a key determinant of population mortality in several studies, starting with the seminal work of Ruhm (2000). Since unemployment rates can change quickly over short periods of time, this information is included in our analysis. For robustness checks, additional information about the population, insurance, and health characteristics is taken from the Area Resource File (ARF).

3.1 Measuring the Geographic Variation of the Impact of Medicare Part D

One of the challenges in this study is to characterize the population that is most affected by Medicare Part D. Intuitively, those individuals most affected by drug insurance expansion should be those who had no drug coverage before the expansion. The institutional features of the insurance market reveal that geography was likely a major source of variation in drug coverage prior to the reform. In particular, two major sources of prescription drug coverage for those age 65 and over before the reform were enrollment in Medicaid or the Medicare Advantage program—both of which varied by geography.

The determinants of the availability of Medicare Advantage (the private insurance alternative) or Medicaid coverage differ substantially. Medicaid eligibility varies greatly by state, where each state determines the exact rules for eligibility in the Medicaid program. The determinants of Medicare Advantage coverage are influenced primarily by private insurers' potential profitability in a particular geographic area. Profitability will depend on a variety of factors, such as the potential number of covered lives in an area (i.e., scale) or the number of insurers offering commercial insurance (i.e., scope), and regulatory considerations (e.g., CMS reimbursement rate). The Medicare regulator, CMS, reimburses Medicare Advantage plans for each covered life. These rates, set by the CMS, vary at the county level, and have been shown to be key determinants of entry across markets.[27] In addition to these sources of geographic variation that are affected by government policy,

---

[27]Regulatory restrictions require that when private insurers enter at the county level they must make plans available to the entire Medicare population in that county. Although Medicare Advantage plans were not required to offer drug benefits before the reform, greater competition in the Medicare Advantage market has been associated with improved generosity of benefits, including drug benefits (Dunn (2011)).

the generosity of retiree benefits, including drug benefits, may vary across regions due to differences in labor market conditions and practices. Geography also plays a major role post-reform, since the private Part D prescription drug insurers choose whether or not to enter each of the 34 regulatory defined regions.

The differences in Part D coverage across the United States reveal the importance of geography. Table 2 shows prescription drug coverage information from the MCBS for the five states most affected by the reform and the five states that appear least affected. There is a large amount of variation across states, with a standard deviation of a 7.9 percent change in drug insurance coverage. There is a clear positive correlation between those lacking drug coverage in a state before the reform and the post-reform gains in coverage.[28]

Table 2: State Level Drug Coverage

State	Pre-Part D (2004-05)	Post-Part D (2006-07)	Change	Obs
Nebraska	31.9%	75.0%	43.1%	365
Arkansas	41.3%	77.5%	36.1%	337
Georgia	46.1%	81.4%	35.2%	1,150
Indiana	52.8%	83.3%	30.4%	118
West Virginia	55.6%	85.9%	30.3%	468
Oklahoma	76.1%	88.3%	12.2%	367
Massachusetts	77.2%	89.0%	11.8%	638
Illinois	69.6%	81.4%	11.8%	1,205
Virginia	71.3%	82.4%	11.1%	443
Arizona	80.8%	90.6%	9.8%	784
Standard Deviation	17.0%	5.1%	13.0%	
p90	78.1%	91.8%	30.3%	
p10	46.9%	76.7%	11.6%	

While Table 2 demonstrates the importance of geographic variation at the state level, the features of the Medicare drug insurance market prior to reform suggest that the effect of Part D should be measured at the county level. However, as can be seen by the number of observations per state over the four-year period, reported in the last column of Table 2, there will be relatively few observations for many counties.

---

[28]It should also be noted that not every state is represented in the MCBS data. The following states have too few observations to be included in the analysis: Alaska, Maine, Idaho, Mississippi, North Dakota, Utah, Oregon, Delaware, New Hampshire, South Dakota, Rhode Island, Vermont, Hawaii, and Montana. See Table D5 for the list of counties used in our main analysis.

In order to capture the variation in prescription drug offerings at the county level, and maximize the accuracy of the county-level estimates, we apply a probit model to predict county-level coverage. Our construction of the predicted change in drug coverage for each county entails a multi-step process. First, we calculate a predicted share of individuals covered in each county before the reform. Next, we repeat this process and calculate a predicted share of individuals covered in each county after the reform. Finally, we calculate the predicted change in drug coverage.

The first step entails running a probit model on the set of individuals in the MCBS prior to the reform. Specifically, we run the following probit on sample years 2004 and 2005 in the MCBS data:

$$\Pr(\text{Covered}_i = 1 | X, \gamma_c) = \Phi(\beta X + \gamma_c), \tag{1}$$

where γ_c are county-specific fixed effects and X is a vector of covariates representing the individual i's age and sex as well as a year dummy.[29] The dependent variable represents an indicator whether individual i has drug coverage.[30] To maximize the accuracy of each county-level estimate, our main estimates use only those counties with at least 30 individual observations over the 2004 to 2005 time period.[31]

We use the population weights from MCBS to derive the predicted pre- and post-reform insurance rate in each county. Specifically, we calculate $SHARE_c^{pre} = \frac{\sum_i w_i \Phi(\hat{\beta} X + \hat{\gamma}_c)}{\sum_i w_i}$ where w_i is a population weight for individual i from the MCBS data, where the weighted means are taken over the entire 2004 and 2005 sample. Essentially, for county c we are computing a coverage rate for the complete distribution of Medicare enrollees pre-reform. Φ represents the normal distribution CDF. We repeat this exercise for individuals for the sample individuals in the 2006 and 2007 MCBS pool, creating a set $SHARE_c^{post}$. The change in insurance coverage in county c is then simply $\Delta INS_c = SHARE_c^{post} - SHARE_c^{pre}$.

There is a considerable amount of variation in this variable. For the 169 counties included in our main sample, the standard deviation of ΔINS_c is 11.3 percent, considerably

---

[29]In our main estimates we include only age and sex information in X, since they are reflected and controlled for in our mortality estimates. Results of this probit estimation are reported in Table D3 of the Appendix. For robustness, we ran a multitude of variations of (1) to calculate the share of covered individuals (e.g., including additional controls in the vector X). See Appendix Table D7.

[30]See Section 3 concerning how we created this drug coverage dummy variable from the MCBS.

[31]See Appendix Table D5 for a list of those counties used in our main analyis. We report results where we lowered this threshold to 15 in Appendix Table D8.

larger than the state-level variation.[32] In addition, this variation appears to match well with prior expectations regarding the underlying cause of across-market pre-reform drug coverage. In particular, Table B1 of the Appendix shows that those counties with higher Medicare Advantage penetration or Medicaid enrollment experienced less of a change in drug coverage as a result of the reform, all else equal. This suggests that using county-level variation is more appropriate for identifying the effects of mortality, relative to broader geographic definitions.

There is some concern that using the measured changes in insurance coverage, ΔINS_c, may be problematic. First, a change in the share of covered individuals in the county may correspond to a change in the health of the population, rather than to Medicare Part D. To address these two issues, we use the insurance coverage *prior* to the reform as a predictor of the change in coverage due to the reform.[33] Figure 4 below shows a scatter plot with a fitted line showing the relationship between the pre-reform level of drug coverage, $SHARE_c^{pre}$ and the percentage change in drug coverage, ΔINS_c, based on the regression $\Delta INS_c = \beta SHARE_c^{pre} + \varepsilon_c$. There is a clear and significant negative relationship and the fit is strong, with an R-squared of 0.89 and a coefficient of -0.83 with standard error of 0.02.

The main specification in our analysis applies the predicted change in insurance, $\widehat{\Delta INS_c}$. That is, $\widehat{\Delta INS_c} = \hat{\beta} SHARE_c^{pre}$.[34] This approach is taken for simplicity, and to more easily translate the effects of the reform on insurance, as predicted by $\widehat{\Delta INS_c}$, to an effect on mortality. However, for completeness we will also present results which apply $SHARE_c^{pre}$

---

[32]See Appendix Table D5 for a list of these counties.

[33]More precisely, Finkelstein (2007) uses the rate of uninsured prior to Medicare's introduction as a measure of the impact of Medicare's change. Since Medicare led to almost full insurance coverage for the 65 and over population, the fraction of individuals uninsured before the reform was equal to the predicted impact of the change. For the Medicare Part D population, the share of individuals without drug insurance is a strong predictor of the change in the share of those insured, but is not equal to the actual change.

[34]Although using solely pre-reform insurance provides a nice fit with the change in coverage, we also explore alternative estimates of predicting the change in drug coverage. For instance, the predicted change may also be calculated using both the pre-insurance level, but also the 34 Medicare Part D geographic regions as a basis for the predicted county-level changes.

Using the Medicare region geography, the predicted change is specified as $\Delta INS_c = \beta SHARE_c^{pre} + \gamma_R + \sum_d (\theta_R \mathbf{D}_R \cdot SHARE_c^{pre}) + \varepsilon_c$ where γ_R are fixed effects for each Medicare Part D region, R. The expression also allows the predicted change in insurance based on the pre-insurance share in each county to vary by region, where $\mathbf{D}$ represents a dummy variable for each Part D region. Thus, this analysis exploits geographic differences in insurance coverage across markets before the reform and also the geography boundaries defined by the reform. Similar results are obtained using either approach.

Figure 4: Regression of Pre-Reform Coverage on Percent Change in Coverage

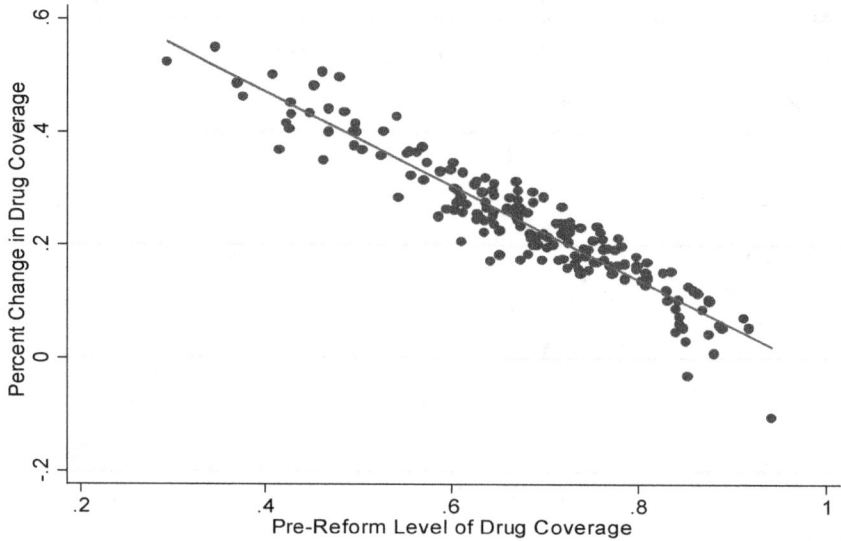

directly.[35]

While our analysis exploits geographic differences in drug coverage, demographic factors may also affect levels of coverage before and after the reform. Specifically, individuals are less likely to have drug coverage as they get older, and this difference is especially large for individuals over the age of 85. There are several reasons that this paper does not focus on demographic variation in insurance coverage as a treatment for policy reform. First, the geographic variation appears to offer considerably more variation, relative to the demographic factors. This may be observed in Table D2 of the Appendix, which shows differences in pre- and post- reform drug coverage by age and sex. Second, much of the demographic variation in prescription drug coverage occurs because of the 85+ population, which is problematic because age adjustment is difficult on this age group. Third, there may be numerous endogeneity concerns, since the level of drug coverage in an area may actually impact the number of individuals that reach the age of 85.[36] Finally, focusing on

[35]Alternatively, one could view the predicted change in insurance as similar to a first stage of a two-stage least squares procedure, where we only use the exogenous pre-reform coverage rates as an instrument. Although this view is not exactly equivalent, we find that applying an instrumental variables estimate on the actual change variable in the regression produces similar results.

[36]For instance, the age categories may be interdependent and introduce noise into the mortality estimates, since an area that has a high mortality rate for 65 to 69-year-olds could later lead to a low mortality rate for 70 to 74-year-olds, if less healthy individuals die before reaching the age of 70. In other words,

geographic variation in coverage simplifies the analysis.[37]

4 Empirical Models

This section first describes a basic difference-in-differences regression model that is used to analyze the effects on mortality. This model will be used to demonstrate many of the key points in this paper. However, we will also note some of the shortcomings and then present an alternative model that views alternative causes of death as competing risks.

4.1 Independent-Risks Model

The basic analysis in this paper focuses on measuring the differential impact of the Part D drug insurance expansion on mortality by applying a linear regression model of mortality that includes county-specific dummies and time-specific dummies to examine the differential change in mortality across counties. The focus will be measuring the predicted change in prescription drug insurance on post-reform mortality. The mortality regression takes the following form:

$$M_{d,t,c} = \tau_d \widehat{\Delta INS}_c \cdot Post_t + \beta_d X_{d,t,c} + \gamma_{d,c} + \gamma_{d,t} + \xi_{d,t,c}, \qquad (2)$$

where $M_{d,t,c}$ is the mortality rate from disease d in year t in county c. The predicted change in drug insurance is $\widehat{\Delta INS}_c$ and $Post_t$ is a dummy variable that equals 1 if the year is 2006 or later. Note that the mortality rate when $t = 2006$ is calculated based on the deaths from mid-2006 to mid-2007, divided by the population in mid-2006. The main parameter to be estimated in this model is τ_d, which captures the effect of the reform on the mortality rate. The county-disease fixed effects are $\gamma_{d,c}$, the year-disease fixed effects are, $\gamma_{d,t}$, and $X_{d,t,c}$ includes additional covariates. We assess two disease-types: $d = \{$cardiovascular, noncardiovascular$\}$ where all deaths fall into one of these two exhaustive categories. The county disease-specific dummies in this analysis are critical because they capture aspects of the population's health in a particular county that are constant both before and after reform. The time dummies are disease specific and account for factors affecting mortality that are the same across all counties, such as common technological progress or information that impacts the treatment of health conditions in all

---

the mortality rates across the age ranges are interrelated.

[37]Additional analysis discussed in Section 6.2.3 allows for the effects of the reform to depend on both geography and demographics and produces similar results. In particular, we allow the predicted change in coverage to depend on the 34 regulatory defined regions.

counties. The variables, $X_{d,t,c}$, may include demographics of the population or the unemployment rate, which has been documented to have a strong correlation with mortality in the literature (see Ruhm (2000)). Additional robustness checks are included that incorporate a variety of information in $X_{d,t,c}$. In equation (2) the disease categories are viewed as independent and estimates for each may be computed using a separate regression for the cardiovascular and noncardiovascular categories. Rather than estimate equation (2) under a single model, we estimate this model under three different samples: cardiovascular mortality, noncardiovascular mortality, and total mortality.[38]

4.2   Competing-Risks Model

While model (2) is simple and intuitive, it also contains some limitations. One issue is that alternative causes of death are interrelated with the mortality rate of other causes. To see this, note that an increase in mortality from cancer necessarily implies a reduction in cardiovascular-related deaths, since those that do not die of cancer eventually die of another cause. This makes it more challenging for model (2) to be used in measuring the effects on total mortality or to think about the role of comorbidities, which are both important measurement issues for studying the effects of mortality. Here we consider a more complete system for measuring mortality by applying a model with three different health states: (1) cardiovascular death, (2) noncardiovascular death, and (3) alive. Following much of the notation of (2), the health state of an individual, i, $h_{d,t,c,i}$, takes the following functional form:

$$h_{d,t,c,i} = \tau_d \widehat{\Delta INS}_c \cdot Post_t + \beta_d X_{d,t,c} + \gamma_{d,c} + \gamma_{d,t} + \xi_{d,t,c} + \epsilon_{d,t,c,i}, \tag{3}$$

where the additional variable contained in (3), $\epsilon_{d,t,c,i}$ includes random factors that determine an individual's cause of death that is not shared by the entire county in time period t. We normalize the health state of being alive to zero. Therefore, the higher the value of the health state variable for cardiovascular-related and noncardiovascular-related conditions, the greater the probability that an individual dies of those respective causes. The main difference under equation (3), relative to the independent-risks model, is that all three options are explicitly viewed as substitutes. For example, if $h_{noncardio,t,c,i} > h_{cardio,t,c,i} > 0$ then a person will die of a noncardiovascular cause, rather than a cardiovascular condition. To provide some structure on the substitution patterns among states, we assume that $\epsilon_{d,t,c,i}$ is independently and identically distributed as type 1 extreme value. Also, let the average

---

[38]The standard errors do not change if the disease categories are estimated separately or jointly.

health of the population in the county for disease d be denoted:

$$\delta_{d,t,c} = \tau_d \widehat{\Delta INS}_c \cdot Post_t + \beta_d X_{d,t,c} + \gamma_{d,c} + \gamma_{d,t} + \xi_{d,t,c}.$$

The usual logit functional form for the shares of individuals dying of disease d in period t is then:

$$s_{d,t,c} = \frac{\exp(\delta_{d,t,c})}{1 + \sum_{d \in \{cardio,noncardio\}} \exp(\delta_{d,t,c})}.$$

Berry (1994) shows that the above model may be estimated with the following linear regression:

$$
\begin{aligned}
\log(s_{d,t,c}) - \log(s_{alive,t,c}) &= \delta_{d,t,c} \\
&= \tau_d \widehat{\Delta INS}_c \cdot Post_t + \beta_d X_{d,t,c} + \gamma_{d,c} + \gamma_{d,t} + \xi_{d,t,c}. \quad (4)
\end{aligned}
$$

Equation 4 provides a simple empirical model, which contains all the potential states of the individual. The model implicitly incorporates the substitution among conditions, where the logit functional form assumes that individuals substitute in proportion to the shares of each health state. One advantage of this approach is it accounts for all health states when measuring the impact on total mortality and it also allows for a clear relationship across alternative causes of death.

Similar to the disease-specific approach, there are two types of mortality rates studied in the competing-risks model. The simple mortality share, $s_{d,t,c}$, considers the share of the population that falls into each of the three health states in each time period. The YLL mortality share, $s_{d,t,c}^{YLL}$, considers the total potential life years in each state at the end of each period. Essentially, this approach weights the population in each age group by the expected years of life for the average individual in that age group. Rather than normalize each county to the 2000 population, this analysis controls for the demographics by including the share of the population in each age-sex category interacted with each condition category as independent variables.[39]

4.2.1 Competing-Risks Model Extensions

The competing-risks model can be extended in a number of ways. In this study, we will perform two extensions. First, we will extend the competing-risks model to incorporate

---

[39]Specifically, the share variables are calculated as: $s_{d,t,c} = \frac{\text{Died}^d_{t \text{ to } t+1}}{\text{Total Population in Period } t}$ and $s_{d,t,c}^{YLL} = \frac{\text{Died}^d_{t \text{ to } t+1} \text{Weighted by Expected Life Years Lost}}{\text{Total Expected Life Years Lost for Population in Period } t}$.

dynamic effects. Second, we will extend the model to account for differential substitution patterns between diseases. We defer discussing the explicit empirical models of both of these extensions until later in the paper. However, below we give an overview of the reasons for including them.

Dynamic Effects

The health of the population in equation (3) is modeled as static, which may be appropriate for the first period of the reform, but could be problematic for measuring the effects on mortality in future periods. As argued in Figure 3, the cardiovascular health of the population in previous periods may influence the health and the mortality rate of a population in subsequent periods.[40] As an extension of our main analysis, we explicitly incorporate these dynamic considerations in the model to study mortality effects over a longer horizon.

Substitution Patterns

A limitation of the basic logit model (4) is that it has restrictive substitution patterns. In particular, the model suffers from the "independence of irrelevant alternatives" problem that is caused by assuming that individuals substitute among alternatives in proportion to the share of each health state. This assumption may be problematic since those who die in period t may have worse health and a greater chance of dying from an alternative cause, compared with the typical individual. In Appendix C, we allow for more flexible substitution patterns by applying a nested-logit model, which is commonly applied in the industrial organization literature using aggregated market share data (Berry (1994)). The nested-logit model will demonstrate the role of substitution patterns when studying mortality data. Most importantly, we show that the results are robust to alternative assumptions regarding substitution patterns among alternative causes of death, which we find to be important in some instances.

5 Independent-Risks Model: Results

In this section, we discuss results using the independent-risks model. We use this framework to tackle two questions. First, we assess the timing of the effect of the reform. Understanding the timing of Part D's effect is critical, since after the initial effect on

---

[40]For example, suppose the reform acts to increase the life expectancy for those with an illness for about one year. In this case, those areas where the reform has a large impact will receive a large reduction in mortality in the amount of $\tau_d \widehat{\Delta INS}_c \cdot Post_t$. However, in the following year the population saved by the reform in the previous year, $\tau_d \widehat{\Delta INS}_c \cdot Post_t$, will include less-healthy individuals who are more likely to die, thereby reducing the health of the population by an amount proportional to $\widehat{\Delta INS}_c \cdot Post_t$.

mortality the subsequent population will include a mix of individuals who are not directly comparable to the pre-Part D population. We use the estimates to inform us about the issues discussed in Figure 3. Second, we use the independent-risks model to measure the effect of the reform in the immediate post-period—the period which contains no delayed-mortality effects. These estimates help inform us about the strength of our identification strategy, but also provide a baseline with which we can compare more complex models later in the study.

5.1 Timing of the Medicare Part D Effect

To investigate the timing of the reform, we begin the analysis of mortality with a more flexible version of equation (2):

$$M_{d,t,c}^{YLL} = \tau_{d,t}\widehat{\Delta INS}_c \cdot \mathbf{D}_t + \beta_d X_{d,t,c} + \gamma_{d,c} + \gamma_{d,t} + \epsilon_{d,t,c}, \tag{5}$$

where we replace the $Post_t$ dummy with flexible time dummies, $\mathbf{D}_t$. It follows that the estimate $\tau_{d,t}$ captures the effect of Part D on mortality for disease-category d in year t. Using this model, the effects of the reform will be measured flexibly in each year both pre- and post-reform.

The estimates of this model are reported in Figure 5, where each year on the x-axis represents the mortality rate from July 1 of the listed year to June 30 of the following year. There are several points to note. First, there are no strong pre-reform trends for either disease category, although we do observe a slight upward trend for noncardiovascular-related mortality and a downward trend in cardiovascular-related mortality in 2005. These trends could potentially represent an initial impact of Part D.[41] One of the striking features in Figure 5 is the effect on cardiovascular-related mortality from July 1, 2006, to June 30, 2007. This sharp and significant drop in cardiovascular-related mortality corresponds precisely to the expected impact of expanding drug coverage. In addition, corresponding to this effect, we also observe a jump in noncardiovascular-related mortalities in the subsequent year. These patterns correspond with the delayed-mortality and competing-risks effects shown in Figure 3. We believe this is a result of a transformation in the health of the population caused by Part D implementation. The immediate timing of the effect

---

[41]Recall that the year 2005 will include the first six months of Part D, which could also be impacted by individuals visiting physicians and purchasing drugs in anticipation of the reform. These trends could also be attributable to the Medicare Discount Drug Card Program (also created by the Medicare Modernization Act) which came into effect in mid-2004. This program was meant to subsidize Medicare recipients for prescription drugs during the two-year period before Part D was fully implemented.

of Part D on mortality is consistent with the finding of Ketcham and Simon (2008) who show that most of the expansion in prescription drug utilization occurred in early 2006. Of course, the patterns in Figure 5 do not match perfectly with those in Figure 3, and there are numerous empirical factors that could cause this divergence. As is common in policy reform studies, many unknown factors may impact measurement as one moves farther from the reform.

Figure 5: Marginal Effect of Predicted Change in Drug Coverage on Mortality

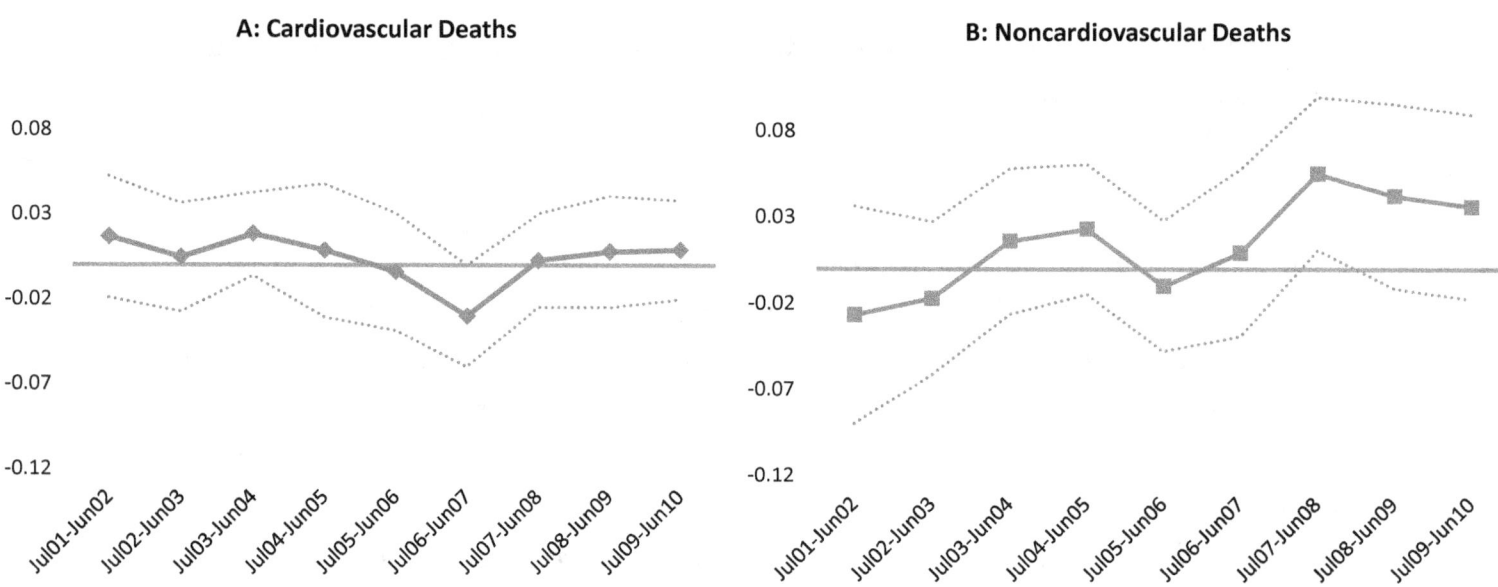

Notes: Red diamonds indicate estimates from specification (5) using cardiovascular mortality as the dependent variable. Blue squares indicate estimates using noncardiovascular mortality as the dependent variable. The omitted year in the regression is 2000 (that is, July 2000 to June 2001). Dotted lines show 95 percent confidence bands. The mortality measure is age-sex adjusted years of life lost for the 65 to 84 population.

Figure 5 highlights the challenges of measuring effects on mortality in the post-reform period. In this setting, identification using a difference-in-differences framework over the entire post-reform period is problematic. County fixed effects, aimed at controlling for the health of the population, will not capture harvesting effects (discussed in Figure 3) as a result of Part D. Indeed, we will show that if dynamic considerations are incorporated into the analysis, then mortality effects of Part D may be identified through 2009. For the basic analysis that follows, which does not incorporate these dynamic effects, we concentrate on

28

the effects on mortality rate measured from mid-2006 to mid-2007.

There are a few additional points to note regarding Figure 5. A decline in mortality of one type appears to be related to an increase in mortality from other causes, as expected. This pattern suggests that a model that explicitly addresses these alternatives in a single competing-risks framework may be useful. Finally, since 2005 includes the first six months in which Part D is implemented, (i.e., January 1st 2006 to July 31st), we drop that year from most of our subsequent analysis.[42]

5.2 Immediate Post-Period Effect of Medicare Part D

To more precisely estimate the effects of the reform, this subsection focuses on mortality effects in the July 1, 2006, to June 30, 2007 period relative to the patterns observed pre-reform. Throughout much of the analysis we examine two different pre-reform periods. One pre-reform period includes all pre-reform periods in our data from 2000-04. The advantage of this approach is that it contains more pre-reform control periods for each county, so more observations are used in determining the baseline mortality rate in each area for each disease. The other pre-reform period uses only 2003-04 as the control years, which includes the mortality rates of the population immediately before the reform. Although this period includes less data to establish baseline mortality rates in each county, it is likely the most comparable to the population immediately after the reform.

Table 3 reports results based on age-sex adjusted years-of-life lost for the age 65 to 84 population.[43] The first three columns show results for those dying from any disease. It appears that there is evidence of the effect of the reform when looking at overall mortality data. Next, we examine the effects of the reform on the two disease categories separately. Recall that this is a more informative estimate that tests a more precisely defined hypothesis. The interpretation of the cardiology coefficient for this specification is that a county that goes from no drug insurance to full drug insurance will have a 0.04 to 0.05 percent reduction in the years of the potential lives lost due to a cardiovascular disease. The mean value of this dependent variable in 2004 is 0.119, so this implies about a 33 percent reduction in cardiovascular-related years of life lost for a hypothetical county that goes from no insurance to full insurance.[44]

---

[42]The year 2005 is also likely affected by the Medicare Discount Drug Card Program. The results are typically very similar when 2005 is included.

[43]In the Appendix, we report results based on mortality rates as well as for all individuals over age 65.

[44]The reduction in the mortality *rate* (in terms of lives, not in terms of years of life lost), shown in Appendix Table D4, is 0.3 to 0.4 percentage points, which is about a 15 percent decline in the mortality rate. In 2004 the mortality rate for cardiovascular disease for the over 65 population was 0.0196, so the

Table 3: Effect of Predicted Change in Drug Insurance on Mortality by Primary Cause of Death

	Overall			Cardiovascular			Noncardiovascular		
Change*Post	-0.061***	-0.041**	-0.065**	-0.037***	-0.040***	-0.050***	-0.023	-0.001	-0.016
	(0.021)	(0.018)	(0.032)	(0.012)	(0.011)	(0.018)	(0.017)	(0.015)	(0.024)
Observations	507	1014	1014	507	1014	1014	507	1014	1014
Sample Years	2003-04, 2006	2000-04, 2006	2000-04, 2006	2003-04, 2006	2000-04, 2006	2000-04, 2006	2003-04, 2006	2000-04, 2006	2000-04, 2006
County Specific Trend	No	No	Yes	No	No	Yes	No	No	Yes

Notes: The mortality measure used in the above estimates is based on the age-sex adjusted years-of-life lost for the age 65 to 84 population. Estimates using alternative measures of mortality are available in Appendix Table D4. Overall mortality includes individuals who died from any cause. Cardiovascular mortality includes only individuals who died from a cardiovascular-related disease as the primary cause of death. noncardiovascular mortality includes only individuals who died from a noncardiovascular-related disease as the primary cause of death. *Post* indicates a post-reform dummy. All regressions include county fixed effects, year dummies, the age distribution of the population, and the unemployment rate. Standard errors clustered by county. $^*p < 0.10$, $^{**}p < 0.05$, $^{***}p < 0.01$.

Table 3 uses the predicted change in drug insurance in the area. Recall that the predicted change is applied, since the actual change is potentially endogenous. However, the key identification stems from the underlying variation in pre-reform differences in drug coverage across geographic markets. To emphasize this point, all of the estimates in Table 3 are repeated in Table 4, but the pre-reform share of the population *without* drug insurance is used instead of the predicted change in drug insurance variable. All the results of Table 4 parallel the results of Table 3 and show that cardiovascular mortality declines are greatest in those counties that had a high share of individuals without drug coverage prior to the reform.

The difference-in-differences analysis in Tables 3 and 4 offers strong evidence that Part D led to a sharp reduction in cardiovascular-related deaths, and the observation that we find no effect on noncardiovascular deaths bolsters this evidence. However, one may be concerned that these patterns could be caused by other health, economic or environmental factors that happen to affect those counties where Part D expansion had the greatest effect. To address this concern we implement a falsification exercise using the population aged 55-64. In particular, if there are other county-disease-specific factors affecting mortality that are unrelated to Part D, we would expect that these factors would also impact the

percentage decline for gaining full insurance is 0.003/0.0196=0.15.

Table 4: Effect of Pre-Part D Coverage on Mortality by Primary Cause of Death

	Overall			Cardiovascular			Noncardiovascular		
(1-CoverageShare)*Post	-0.050***	-0.033**	-0.054**	-0.031***	-0.033***	-0.041***	-0.019	-0.001	-0.013
	(0.017)	(0.015)	(0.027)	(0.010)	(0.009)	(0.015)	(0.014)	(0.012)	(0.020)
Observations	507	1014	1014	507	1014	1014	507	1014	1014
Sample Years	2003-04, 2006	2000-04, 2006	2000-04, 2006	2003-04, 2006	2000-04, 2006	2000-04, 2006	2003-04, 2006	2000-04, 2006	2000-04, 2006
County Specific Trend	No	No	Yes	No	No	Yes	No	No	Yes

Notes: The mortality measure used in the above estimates is based on the age-sex adjusted years-of-life lost for the age 65 to 84 population. Overall mortality includes individuals who died from any cause. Cardiovascular mortality includes only individuals who died from a cardiovascular related disease as the primary cause of death. noncardiovascular mortality includes only individuals who died from a noncardiovascular-related disease as the primary cause of death. *Post* indicates a post-reform dummy. All regressions include county fixed effects, year dummies, the age distribution of the population, and the unemployment rate. Standard errors clustered by county. $*p < 0.10$, $**p < 0.05$, $***p < 0.01$.

55-64 aged population. Table 5 presents results of this exercise, which show no statistically significant effect on the below 65 population. As another falsification exercise, we implement a "triple" difference-in-differences specification, where we assess both the age 55 to 64 population and the 65 to 84 population in the same regression. The results are reported in Table 6. We find that the 65+ population has a negative and significant reduction in cardiovascular- related deaths post-reform relative to the effects on the 55-64 population, within the same county. This result offers even stronger evidence that the reform led to a reduction in cardiovascular-related deaths for the 65+ population.

Although we find a significant difference across the older and younger populations, we focus primarily on the 65 and over population in the remainder of the analysis. The main reason is that the within-Medicare 55-64 population is relatively less healthy. Since insurance information is not available in the CDC mortality data, the effects on the 55-64 Medicare population cannot be cleanly identified. As mentioned earlier, there is also a potential for spillover effects across populations. For example, younger populations may take more prescription drugs simply because older individuals who live nearby are taking prescription drugs.

Table 5: Effect of Predicted Change in Drug Insurance on Mortality by Primary Cause of Death: Age 55-64 Population

	Cardiovascular			Noncardiovascular		
Change*Post	-0.013	-0.010	-0.018	-0.005	0.008	-0.036
	(0.011)	(0.010)	(0.023)	(0.024)	(0.021)	(0.038)
Observations	507	1014	1014	507	1014	1014
Sample Years	2003-04, 2006	2000-04, 2006	2000-04, 2006	2003-04, 2006	2000-04, 2006	2000-04, 2006
County Specific Trend	No	No	Yes	No	No	Yes

Notes: The mortality measures used in the above estimates are based on the age-sex adjusted years-of-life lost for the age 55 to 64 population. Cardiovascular mortality includes only individuals who died from a cardiovascular-related disease as the primary cause of death. noncardiovascular mortality includes only individuals who died from a noncardiovascular related disease as the primary cause of death. *Post* indicates a post-reform dummy. All regressions include county fixed effects, year dummies, the age distribution of the population and the unemployment rate. Standard errors clustered by county. $^{*}p < 0.10$, $^{**}p < 0.05$, $^{***}p < 0.01$.

6 Competing-Risks Model: Results

We now turn to measuring the effects of Part D on mortality by applying the competing-risks model. The results of the competing-risks model are similar to the independent-risks model. This is reflected in the results reported in Table 7. Column (1) reports results using only 2003-04 as the pre-period, while the specification in column (2) uses the entire 2000-04 period. The results across both estimates are as expected, a negative and significant drop in cardiovascular-related deaths. The effect on noncardiovascular deaths is small and statistically insignificant.

One alternative hypothesis is that, prior to reform, the health and mortality trends may be different in those counties most impacted by the reform relative to those counties that are less affected. To investigate this issue, in column (3) we include county-specific mortality trends that are common across the two disease categories. This specification is quite flexible as it allows for the health of the population to decline in some counties, but improve in others. Even after incorporating these flexible trends, the estimates in column (3) look very similar to those in columns (1) and (2). Although this specification is flexible, one may be concerned that column (3) is not flexible enough. For example, cardiovascular-related mortality may be declining relative to noncardiovascular mortality in those counties most impacted by the reform. In other words, there may be disease-specific trends that are affecting these patterns. To introduce additional flexibility, we

Table 6: Effect of Predicted Change in Drug Insurance on Mortality by Primary Cause of Death: Triple Difference-in-Differences with Age 55-64 and 65-84 Populations

	Cardiovascular			Noncardiovascular		
Change*Post*$D_{Age \geq 65}$	-0.019	-0.029**	-0.035**	-0.018	-0.013	-0.009
	(0.018)	(0.014)	(0.015)	(0.031)	(0.024)	(0.028)
Change*Post	-0.013	-0.010	-0.013	-0.005	0.010	-0.026
	(0.012)	(0.011)	(0.018)	(0.024)	(0.021)	(0.029)
Observations	1014	2028	2028	1014	2028	2028
Sample Years	2003-04, 2006	2000-04, 2006	2000-04, 2006	2003-04, 2006	2000-04, 2006	2000-04, 2006
County Specific Trend	No	No	Yes	No	No	Yes

Notes: The mortality measures used in the above estimates are based on the age-sex adjusted years-of-life lost for the age 55 to 64 population. Cardiovascular mortality includes only individuals who died from a cardiovascular related disease as the primary cause of death. noncardiovascular mortality includes only individuals who died from a noncardiovascular related disease as the primary cause of death. *Post* indicates a post-reform dummy. All regressions include county fixed effects, year dummies, the age distribution of the population and the unemployment rate. Standard errors clustered by county. $*p < 0.10$, $**p < 0.05$, $***p < 0.01$.

allow for unique mortality trends in each county by disease-category. The results with the county-disease specific trend are presented in column (4). Again, the results barely change from the estimates in columns (1) and (2), although the statistical significance declines, likely due to the loss in degrees of freedom.

The estimates from column (1) imply that a 1 percentage point increase in the share of the population with drug insurance leads to an average 0.0030 percent reduction in years of life lost. That is, for 100,000 years of potential life years lived, a 1 percentage point increase in prescription drug coverage would save three life years. For all estimates, we find that mortality rates for cardiovascular-related conditions significantly decline and so does overall mortality, tested by applying a Wald test of the joint significance of $\tau_{cardio} + \tau_{noncardio}$.[45]

This section does not present results for the below-65 population. However, in a separate analysis we estimated a model using the logit framework using the under-65 population as a control group. We found the results to be qualitatively very similar to those reported in Table 5.

---

[45] As an alternative, the significant effect on mortality is also tested by bootstrapping the marginal effect of drug insurance expansion on mortality, where the standard errors are computed using a sample that clusters at the county level and similar results are found.

Table 7: Logit Competing-Risks Model: Effect of Predicted Change in Drug Insurance on Mortality

	(1)	(2)	(3)	(4)
Change*Post*Cardio	-0.216***	-0.223***	-0.296***	-0.291**
	(0.080)	(0.083)	(0.087)	(0.116)
Change*Post*NonCardio	-0.067	0.019	-0.054	-0.059
	(0.063)	(0.056)	(0.095)	(0.086)
Observations	1014	2028	2028	2028
Sample Years	2003-04, 2006	2000-04, 2006	2000-04, 2006	2000-04, 2006
County-Disease FE	Yes	Yes	Yes	Yes
County Specific Trend	No	No	Yes	No
County-Disease Specific Trend	No	No	No	Yes

Notes: The mortality share measures used in the above estimates are based on the years-of-life lost for the age 65 to 84 population. Estimates using the actual mortality shares are available in Appendix Table D6. Robustness tests are available in Appendix Table D8. All regressions include county-disease fixed effects, year-disease fixed effects, the age distribution of the population, and the unemployment rate. Standard errors clustered by county. $*p < 0.10$, $**p < 0.05$, $***p < 0.01$.

6.1 Incorporating Dynamic Effects

The previous analysis measured the effect on mortality exactly when Part D was implemented, which may not reflect mortality effects in subsequent periods. As argued throughout this paper, this approach was taken purposefully, since the impact of the reform should be expected to change the health of the population, which will complicate the measurement of mortality in future periods. The primary issue is that measuring the effects of Part D in future periods must take into account the impact of the reform on the health of the population in subsequent periods. This subsection attempts to address this issue.

Importantly, the lag of the dependent variable contains information regarding the changing health of the population. If a relatively small fraction of individuals die from cardiovascular-related diseases in a previous period, relative to the average amount for that county, this likely implies a relatively large stock of individuals in the population who may suffer or die from this illness in a subsequent period. The lag of the dependent variable may be incorporated into the empirical model to capture changes in the health of the population, as well as changes in the health of the population related to the reform. Let the lag of the dependent variable be denoted $\delta_{d,t-1,c}$. The model that incorporates these dynamic considerations is the following:

$$
\begin{aligned}
\delta_{d,t,c} \;=\;& \tau_d \widehat{\Delta INS}_c \cdot Post_t + \beta X_{d,t,c} && (6)\\
&+ [\kappa_{d,1}\delta_{d,t-1,c} + \kappa_{d,2}\delta_{d,t-1,c}\widehat{\Delta INS}_c \cdot Post_{t-1}\\
&+ \kappa_{d,3}\delta_{d,t-1,c}\widehat{\Delta INS}_c + \kappa_{d,4}\delta_{d,t-1,c} \cdot Post_{t-1}]\\
&+ \gamma_{d,c} + \gamma_{d,t} + \xi_{d,t,c},
\end{aligned}
$$

where the dynamic terms are included in the bracketed expression. The term $\delta_{d,t-1,c}$ captures the health of the population in the previous period for disease d, and its systematic relationship to current period mortality. The model also allows for the lagged dependent variable to have a unique effect one period after the reform, which is proportional to the magnitude of the reform's effect, through the expression $\delta_{d,t-1,c}\widehat{\Delta INS}_c Post_{t-1}$ where the term $Post_{t-1}$ is an indicator if the year is 2007 or later (i.e., one year after the reform). This second expression is crucial, since it is likely that many individuals changed treatment as a result of the reform, resulting in a change in survival in subsequent periods in proportion to those affected by the Part D introduction. For completeness, two additional terms are added. The term $\delta_{d,t-1,c}\widehat{\Delta INS}_c$ allows for the dynamic relationship to be different over the entire sample period for those counties predicted to be most impacted by the reform. Another term, $\delta_{d,t-1,c}Post_{t-1}$, captures the change in this dynamic relationship across all counties one year after the reform.

Table 8 reports the results of the analysis where the full sample from 2001-2009 is studied.[46] Excluding the lag terms, shown in column (1), there is no effect of Part D on cardiovascular-related deaths, and the results even show a significant increase in noncardiovascular-related deaths. The model in column (2) includes the additional lagged dependent-variable terms. The change in the results is striking, with the effect of Part D having a negative and statistically significant effect on cardiovascular post-reform mortality, while the effect on noncardiovascular mortality becomes insignificant. As one might expect from our analysis depicted in Figure 5, the coefficient on the lagged-dependent variable interacted with the Part D change, $\kappa_{d,2}$, shows that for those counties most impacted by the reform, a drop in mortality post-reform has a statistically significant increase in

---

[46] The year 2000 is dropped since equation 6 contains a lag. In the estimates the year 2005 is excluded since it is a transition period, but the estimates remain unchanged if this year is included. The full sample is studied here, since many observations are necessary to capture the systematic relationship between the current and lagged dependent variables. Robustness tests are available in Appendix Table D9.

Table 8: Logit Competing-Risks Model: Effect of Predicted Change in Drug Insurance on Mortality with Dynamic Considerations

	(1)	(2)
Change*Cardio*Post$_t$	0.052	-0.315***
	(0.056)	(0.077)
Change*NonCardio*Post$_t$	0.103**	-0.016
	(0.044)	(0.062)
Change*Cardio*Post$_{t-1}$*$\delta_{cardio,t-1}$		-0.063***
		(0.020)
Change*NonCardio*Post$_{t-1}$*$\delta_{noncardio,t-1}$		-0.029**
		(0.014)
Cardio*Post$_{t-1}$*$\delta_{cardio,t-1}$		0.041
		(0.033)
NonCardio*Post$_{t-1}$*$\delta_{noncardio,t-1}$		0.064*
		(0.037)
Change*Cardio*$\delta_{cardio,t-1}$		-0.580**
		(0.245)
Change*NonCardio*$\delta_{noncardio,t-1}$		-0.621
		(0.401)
Cardio*$\delta_{cardio,t-1}$		0.110
		(0.085)
NonCardio*$\delta_{noncardio,t-1}$		0.014
		(0.153)
Observations	2704	2704
Sample Years	2001-04, 2006-09	2001-04, 2006-09

Notes: The share measures used in the above estimates are based on the years-of-life lost for the 65 to 84 population. Robustness tests are available in Appendix Table D9. All regressions include county-disease fixed effects, year-disease fixed effects, the age distribution of the population, and the unemployment rate. Standard errors clustered by county. $^*p < 0.10$, $^{**}p < 0.05$, $^{***}p < 0.01$.

the mortality rate in the following period. That is, this term provides evidence of the dynamic effects of the reform. It is also interesting to note that the magnitude of the secondary effect is considerably smaller than the initial impact of the reform, leading to a net reduction in the cardiovascular-related mortality rate in all subsequent periods.[47]

One issue with applying equation (6) is that it incorporates both fixed effects and lagged dependent variables in the model. When the number of time periods is small, this estimation strategy potentially leads to inconsistent estimates (see Nickell (1981)). The concern arises because the change in the lagged-dependent variable is necessarily related to the change in the error term, $\xi_{d,t,c}$. However, we tested the model for serial correlation

---

[47]Similar effects are found if the sample is only extended to 2007 or 2008.

in the error term using the Wooldridge test (Drukker (2003)) and found strong evidence that this was not impacting our results.[48]

The results of Table 8 indicate that the mortality effects of Part D continue through our entire sample. The results in Table 8 also confirm the intuition described in Figure 3. Specifically, once the change in the health of the population post-reform is accounted for, through $\kappa_{d,2}$, the effects on mortality hold throughout the entire sample. While this result supports the previous results, as with all studies of policy effects, there are more factors that could explain the effects of reform on mortality as one moves farther away from the event, leading to less precise estimates.

An important result in Table 8 is the statistically significant *increase* in noncardiovascular-related deaths, reported in column (1). While this result may appear counterintuitive, it fits a competing-risks framework where individuals saved from one illness are more likely to die from a competing risk in a future period. This is highlighted by the fact that after including controls for the changing health of the population, we see this relationship disappear. The nested logit analysis, discussed below as part of our robustness analysis, further reinforces this point by capturing a strong correlation among alternative causes of death.

6.2   Robustness Analysis

6.2.1   nested logit Model

As an alternative specification, we estimate a model that incorporates more complex substitution patterns— a nested logit model. The nested logit specification is important if there is strong substitution among alternative causes of death caused by many individuals in the population having comorbidities. The logit functional form assumes that substitution between causes of death is in proportion to shares. Since "alive" represents a large share of the health state in each market, substitution toward the health state of "alive" is likely overstated and substitution to noncardiovascular deaths is understated. Since the substitution to alternative causes of death is not reflected in the model, the effect of Part D on mortality may show up as both a negative effect on cardiovascular mortality, but also a positive bias on noncardiovascular mortality. This pattern could lead to a mistaken

---

[48]Specifically, the p-value on the F-statistic testing the null-hypothesis of no serial correlation on equation (4) under the 2000 to 2009 sample was 0.80. We also performed a robustness exercise in which we removed the county-disease fixed effects and included the year 2000 value of the dependent variable as a control. No results changed.

conclusion regarding the effects of the reform.

The results of this exercise are described in Appendix C. For our nested logit model, we add a third type of mortality category that includes individuals who die of a noncardiovascular illness, who are recorded as having a cardiovascular comorbidity at the time of their death. The model allows for a distinct correlation pattern among those individuals who die from a cardiovascular illness or have a cardiovascular comorbidity. We find a strong correlation between individuals who die of cardiovascular-related causes and those who die of other causes but have a cardiovascular comorbidity. As one might expect, when we do not account for the correlation among alternative causes of death we tend to find a positive effect of the reform on those that have a cardiovascular comorbidity, but die of alternative cause. This effect disappears when we allow for stronger correlation among these alternative causes of death. Importantly, we find the main result is robust to this alternative specification, showing a significant decline in cardivascular related deaths across all specifications.

6.2.2 Instrumental Variables

To gain a better understanding of some of the sources of geographic variation in pre-reform drug coverage, we assessed an instrumental-variables specification of the competing-risks model. This analysis is shown in Appendix B. First, we show that those areas where Medicare Advantage and Medicaid penetration were higher prior to the reform, experienced less drug insurance expansion post reform. We find that using variation in Medicaid and Medicare Advantage enrollment rates prior to the reform as instruments results in mortality effects similar to our main analysis. In other words, exploiting only the change in drug coverage related to Medicaid and Medicare Advantage market penetration prior to the reform, we still find that Part D expansion affects mortality. This alternative source of identification is reassuring, since both Medicaid and Medicare Advantage programs are impacted greatly by exogenous policies and market conditions.

6.2.3 Additional Robustness Checks

To check the robustness of our results, we performed a multitude of alternative specifications. Appendix Table D8 shows estimates of specification (4) under alternative samples, weighting, and age cutoffs for the mortality measure. Appendix Table D7 shows estimates under alternative specifications and time periods to construct $SHARE_c^{pre}$ and $SHARE_c^{post}$. Additional robustness checks have also been conducted, such as removing states that may be impacted by Hurricane Katrina.[49] The main findings hold across all of these additional checks.

A potential critique of our analysis is that it focuses only on the *geographic* differences in prescription drug coverage across areas. Demographic differences may also affect how individuals are impacted by the reform. As mentioned previously, allowing the effect of Part D to differ by both geography and demographics was not used for a variety of reasons. To assess the robustness of our results, we conduct additional analysis that makes a predicted change in drug coverage from the reform based on both geographic and demographic factors, available in column (5) of Table D7 in Appendix D. Specifically, we estimate a probit model that includes county fixed effects, along with dummies for age (i.e., above and below 75), sex, and age-sex interactions for each of the nine Census divisions. A unique prediction of the change in coverage attributable to Part D is created for each age-sex category in each county, greatly increasing the number of predicted change observations. The mortality data are then constructed to match the county-disease-age-sex categories, so that there are eight mortality estimates for each county (i.e., (above or below 75)*(male or female)*(cardiovascular or noncardiovascular)). The analysis includes many additional fixed effects, with a separate fixed effect for each county-disease-age-sex category. The results lie in the range of the estimates reported in the text. These estimates demonstrate that controlling for the impact of Part D by geography and demographics has little effect on the main results.

7 Measuring the Value of Medicare Part D Expansion

In this section, we compare the implied change in expenditures attributable to the reform to the gains in lives saved by reform. To do so requires us to first estimate the causal impact of the reform on drug expenditures. We then use these estimates to construct cost estimates of the reform in 2007, which are then compared with the value of lives saved in 2007.

---

[49]The eight states most impacted by Katrina, either directly or indirectly through migration, include Texas, Arkansas, Louisiana, Mississippi, Alabama, Tennessee, Georgia, and Florida. See http://seer.cancer.gov/data/hurricane.html.

7.1 Measuring the Effect of Part D on Expenditures

In addition to showing the effects of Part D on mortality, we will show that Part D has the expected effects on prescription drug expenditures. This is, a necessary step in establishing the causal relationship that we are measuring. We measure these effects using the individual-level information from the MCBS survey on total prescription drug expenditures. Specifically, total prescription drug expenditures for individual i will be measured as a function of the policy change, county fixed effects, time dummies, and numerous individual characteristics. Due to the skewness of the data and observations with zero expenditures, the model will be estimated using a GLM model with a log-link.[50] The following is the functional form of the GLM model:

$$E_{i,t,c} = \exp(\tau \widehat{\Delta INS}_c \cdot Post_t + \beta Z_{i,t,c} + \gamma_c + \gamma_t) + v_{i,t,c}. \tag{7}$$

Many of the elements of this model follow the analysis of mortality, since the data include county fixed effects, α_c, time fixed effects, γ_t, and the predicted impact of the introduction of Part D is captured using the predicted change in drug insurance coverage. The term $v_{i,t,c}$ represents a random error term.[51]

Similarly, we can evaluate the expected change of Part D on out-of-pocket costs. Specifically, let the out-of-pocket expenditure share for individual i be the ratio: $\frac{oopc_{i,t,c}}{E_{i,t,c}}$.[52] We then estimate the effect of the reform using the following log-linear model:

$$\log(\frac{oopc_{i,t,c}}{E_{i,t,c}}) = \tau \widehat{\Delta INS}_c \cdot Post_t + \beta Z_{i,t,c} + \gamma_c + \gamma_t + w_{i,t,c}. \tag{8}$$

Using the predictions from equation (7) and equation (8) on the Medicare population, one can compute the total impact of the reform on total expenditures and out-of-pocket costs. In addition to confirming that Part D has the expected effects on these variables,

---

[50]We explore the impact of alternative functional forms, and obtain similar elasticities across alternative specifications.

[51]The price of the underlying drugs are not likely to play an important role in this specification because drugs are often negotiated on a national level, so the average effect on negotiated prices will be captured by γ_t. However, to the extent that those with insurance pay a lower price than those without, the expenditure effect will include those price differences, so the expenditure change will understate the full quantity response (see Duggan and Morton (2010) for additional details relating to Part D's effect on prices).

[52]In cases where expenditure information is not observed, we use characteristics of the individual, such as insurance plan information, county location, year, and demographics to predict the expected out-of-pocket cost for each individual. We find similar estimates when we use these imputed values and when we do not.

evaluating the effect of the reform on total expenditures is important, as this will assist in determining the cost effectiveness of this spending. By computing both the impact on the expenditures and out-of-pocket expenditure share, these two measures may be used to calculate a price elasticity of demand, which may be benchmarked to other estimates in the literature. Alternatively, equation (7) may be adapted to estimate the price-elasticity of demand for prescription drugs directly by including the out-of-pocket expenditure share for the individual and instrumenting using the Part D policy change. This individual level demand estimation is discussed in greater detail in Appendix A.[53]

The first column of Table 9 reports the results that look at the relationship between the predicted change in prescription drug insurance in the county and the effects on individual drug expenditures (i.e., equation (7)). The effect of Part D on expenditures is positive and significant. We explore alternative functional forms and specifications, but all of the estimates have a coefficient near 0.41. In this case, a 10 percent point change in the share of individuals with insurance, implies a 4.1 percent increase in expenditures. We use these estimates to run a counterfactual in each county that compares the expected change in expenditure with the expected change in expenditure when there is no policy change. Based on these estimates and applying population weights from the MCBS data, we find that the expected expenditures increase by 10 percent over the scenario with no reform.[54]

Next we turn to the effects of the reform on the share of expenditures paid out-of-pocket (i.e., equation (8)). Specifically, the dependent variable is $\log\left(\frac{\text{out-of-pocket expenditures}}{\text{total medical expenditures}}\right)$. We find the out-of-pocket share data to be much less skewed, so we estimate the effects of the reform by applying an ordinary least squares regression model, reported in column (2). Based on these estimates, we find a coefficient of -1.51 that is negative and highly significant. The estimate implies a 31 percent reduction in out-of-pocket spending share caused by the Part D reform, changing from a 24 percent expenditure share in 2007 to a

_____

[53]Note that, in contrast to the measurement of mortality, dynamic considerations are likely less important for looking at expenditures for a few reasons. First, individual information about each person's health, reflecting their knowledge about their health condition, is observed in the MCBS survey. This health information is likely a key determinant affecting expenditures. In contrast, mortality is affected by the observed health of the individual, but also factors unknown to the individual. For example, those individuals with less access to health care or prescription drugs may be less aware of their medical conditions. Moreover, mortality rates are determined by a small segment of the population with the worst health, so that the marginal health of the population may change more rapidly from period to period with shocks to the mortality rate. In contrast, drug expenditures are determined by a larger share of the population. For these reasons, we study expenditures over the period 2004-08.

[54]Based on the different model specifications, the counterfactual increases ranged from about 9 percent to 14 percent.

counterfactual estimate of 34 percent with no reform. Together, based on the estimates of expenditure changes and out-of-pocket share changes, we find an arc price elasticity of -0.26, which is similar to the estimates found in the RAND study. A more direct demand estimation approach applying IV techniques and using the Part D change in coverage variable as an instrument, we obtain similar elasticity estimates, centered around -0.20, but ranging from -0.176 to -0.262. The price elasticity of demand estimates implied by these estimates are comparable to those found in the health literature (see Chandra et al. (2010) and the RAND study (Newhouse (1993))). See Appendix A for an analysis of demand that uses the Part D expansion as an instrument to measure the price elasticity of demand at the individual level.

Table 9: Predicted Change in Drug Insurance on Total and Out-of-Pocket Drug Expenditures

	Log(Exp.)	Log(OOP Share)
Change*Post	0.411**	-1.509***
	(0.189)	(0.194)
Observations	31262	30448
Model	GLM, Poisson	OLS, Log-Linear

Notes: All regressions include county and year fixed effects, as well as controls for demographics (i.e. age, sex, race, education, income), BMI, and disease dummies (arteriosclerotic HD, hypertension, acute myocardial infarction, angina, diabetes, and "other heart conditions"). Standard errors clustered by county. $*p < 0.10$, $**p < 0.05$, $***p < 0.01$.

This paper is the first to use geographic differences in Part D effects to measure the impact on drug expenditures, while other work in the literature primarily focuses on the differential expenditures for those above and below 65. Despite the difference in the approach taken here, the magnitude of the estimates fall in the same range as previous estimates in the literature. While some estimates on the effect of utilization are larger than ours (e.g., Lichtenberg and Sun (2007) find Part D increased utilization by 13 percent), others find more modest increases in expenditures (e.g., Ketcham and Simon (2008) find an increase of 8 percent in total prescription-drug spending while Khan and Kaestner (2009) find an increase of 4-10 percent in utilization). As for the impact on out-of-pocket costs, Ketcham and Simon find a more modest decline in out-of-pocket costs of around 17 percent.

7.2   Comparison of Lives Saved to Drug Expenditures Increases

We now incorporate the results on expenditures with the results on mortality. This allows us to monetize the value of lives saved and compare this amount with total expenditures to give a measure of the overall value of the reform. To simplify the analysis, we focus only on 2007.[55] The findings of this analysis are included in Table 10, which includes analysis that is scaled to the overall impact on the 65+ Medicare population.[56]

The top half of Table 10 reports estimates of the reform's effect related to expenditures. The MCBS population weights are applied to arrive at a total expenditure estimate on prescription drugs for 2007 of around $79 billion. The estimated impact of the reform on expenditures, based on estimates from the first column of Table 9, is 10 percent, which amounts to an expenditure increase caused by the reform of $7.9 billion. A back-of-the-envelope calculation is conducted to arrive at expenditure figures for cardiovascular-related conditions. Since about 48 percent of total drug expenditures are on cardiovascular-related drugs, we estimate that the share of additional spending on cardiovascular-related drugs is $3.8 billion (i.e., $7.8·48 percent). Second, to arrive at a figure of out-of-pocket expenditures for prescription drugs, we use the average share of out-of-pocket post-reform spending of 23 percent, to arrive at the total increase in out-of-pocket spending on cardiovascular drugs of $871 million.

Next, we calculate the effects of the reform on lives saved in 2007 and then monetize this amount by assigning $200,000 per statistical life year.[57] One of the models used to analyze the effects on total mortality are the estimates from column (1) of Table 7 that include only the 2003-04 pre-period. The results from the mortality estimates are shown near the bottom of Table 10. For the mortality estimates based on weighting the years of life saved, we calculate an annualized figure of lives saved by computing average number of life-years per person, which is around 12 (i.e., we compute the total life-years saved divided by the total amount of potential life years per person). Dividing the number of life-years saved by 12 provides an approximate estimate of the number of individuals expected to die

---

[55]A more complete analysis would take into account the full dynamics that control for the changing health of the population. However, as argued in the text, we think the measure of the immediate effects on mortality are likely to be more accurate.

[56]Another important point to note is that the geographic coverage is limited by the fact that the MCBS does not cover all states and many counties had too few observations to accurately measure the impact of Part D. However, the estimates from the counties actually used in the analysis is scaled to the 2007 figures for the entire U.S.

[57]This is the amount applied in Eggleston et al. (2011).

Table 10: Cost-Benefit Analysis of Part D Expansion in 2007

Cost Estimates

1. Population in 2007 Over 65 (in millions) (MCBS)	34.53
2. Total Drugs Expenditures in 2007 (in millions) (MCBS)	$78,863
3. Expenditures Per Capita ((line 2)/(line 1))	$2,284
4. Growth in the Number of Individuals with Drug Insurance (in millions)*	6.22
5. Expenditure Growth Caused by Reform (in millions)*	$7,886
6. Total Exp. on Cardio Conditions (approx 48% of total) (in millions)**	$3,785
7. Additional Out-of-pocket Expenditures (approx 23% of Cardio total) (in millions)***	$871

Benefit Estimates For Lives Saved

Mortality Estimates - Table 6, Column (1)

8. Total Lives Saved (in thousands)	19.3
9. Total Expenditure Per Life Saved - $200,000 per life year (in millions)	$3,865

Mortality Estimates - Table 6, Column (4) - Trend

10. Total Lives Saved (in thousands)	27.1
11. Total Benefits From Lives Saved - $200,000 per life year (in millions)	$5,423

Mortality Estimates - Table 7, Column (2)

12. Total Lives Saved (in thousands)	19.5
13. Total Annual Benefits From Lives Saved - $200,000 per life year (in millions)	$3,900

Notes: *Amount is computed based on predicted change from Part D for those counties with 30 or more observations, but applying the amount to the full population. The drug insurance definition includes additional individuals receiving drug insurance, where the definition of drug insurance depends on the generosity of the plan. Predicted expenditure growth is based on the Poisson estimates in Table 9.

**Calculated as a share of cardiovascular drug expenditures over the period 2003-09 from the underlying MEPS data.

***Applying the observed ratio of out-of-pocket expenditures for drugs to total drug expenditures from Table 1.

within the year.[58] Estimates based on two other specifications are also reported. One is based on estimates including disease-county trends, column (4) of Table 7, and the other is based on the dynamic estimates, column (2) of Table 8. The number of lives saved ranges from 19,000 to 27,000. In dollar terms this amounts to between $3.9 and $5.4 billion in the value of lives saved.

The estimated value of lives saved greatly exceeds the out-of-pocket expenditures of individuals on cardiovascular drugs, which is consistent with individuals purchasing prescription drugs whose benefit exceeds the out-of-pocket costs. What is surprising is that the value of the additional drugs purchased for our preferred specifications ($3.9 to $5.4 billion) exceeds the total cost of the drugs ($3.8 billion). Even using a smaller monetized value of a statistical life, say $100,000, produces sizable gains of over $1.9 billion.

The analysis here does not consider the welfare benefits of reducing the financial risk of the population. The work of Engelhardt and Gruber (2011) examine this issue and find that the welfare benefits of financial protection are about $455 per beneficiary, on average, or $15.7 billion in total.[59] This amount is slightly larger than the deadweight loss that they estimate of $430 per recipient, or $14.8 billion. Incorporating the health benefits of cardiovascular treatments into the calculation adds between $112-$157 in welfare benefits per Medicare beneficiary, suggesting an overall welfare gain from Part D's introduction of at least $137 per beneficiary or $4.7 billion per year.

8   Conclusion

This paper examines the impact of the Part D prescription drug insurance expansion on mortality for the above-65 population. Applying a difference-in-differences framework that exploits the geographic differences in drug coverage across markets prior to reform, we find a statistically significant reduction in cardiovascular-related deaths, saving between 19,000 and 27,000 lives in its first year. While the exact magnitude of the number of lives saved depends on the particular specification, the basic result of a decline in cardiovascular-related deaths is shown to hold up across a multitude of robustness tests.

We find two key features of the analysis that are critical for identifying the effects

---

[58]Using the actual number of years of life saved is likely to greatly overestimate lives saved, since those individuals who are saved tend to be less healthy than average and are less likely to live the expected number of years, as expressed in the life tables. In addition, to make the years of life saved line up with the expenditure figures, we would need to calculate expenditures for all future years.

[59]We are scaling up to the number of Medicare individuals over 65 in the MCBS data

from the Part D program. First, we recognize that the Part D reform may transform the health of the population in future periods. Consequently, much of our analysis focuses on the impact of the reform immediately after implementation. Second, we study the impact of mortality on the condition that is most likely to be impacted by the reform, cardiovascular-related conditions.

It is unclear whether the insights applied in this paper to measure the effects of Part D reform would be effective in measuring the impact of policy changes on mortality in other settings. Indeed, it may be that the unique features of the Part D insurance expansion may have led to identifiable effects on mortality (e.g., proven and effective drugs for treating cardiovascular conditions). However, we hope that the basic lessons learned in this study may lead to new insights for studying the effects of reforms on mortality across other settings.

References

[1] Antithrombotic Trialists' Collaboration, (2002), "Collaborative meta-analysis of randomized trials of antiplatelet therapy for prevention of death, myocardial infarction, and stroke in high risk patients," *BMJ*, 324(7329) pgs 71-86.

[2] Berry, Steven, (1994), "Estimating Discrete-Choice Models of Product Differentiation," *Rand Journal of Economics*, 25, pgs 242-262.

[3] Berry, Steven, James Levinsohn, and Ariel Pakes, (2004), "Differentiated Products Demand Systems from a Combination of Micro and Macro Data: The New Car Market," *Journal of Political Economy*, 112(1), pgs 68-105.

[4] Baicker, Katherine, Sarah Taubman, Heidi Allen, Mira Bernstein, Jonathan Gruber, Joseph Newhouse, Eric Schneider, Bill Wright, Alan Zaslavsky, and Amy Finkelstein, (2013), "The Oregon Experiment - Effects of Medicaid on Clinical Outcomes," *New England Journal of Medicine*.

[5] Blood Pressure Lowering Treatment Trialists' Collaboration. 2003. "Effects of different blood-pressure-lowering regimens on major cardiovascular events: results of prospectively-designed overviews of randomised trials." *Lancet* Vol. 362. pgs 1527-35.

[6] Card, David, Carlos Dobkin, Nicole Maestas, (2009), "Does Medicare Save Lives?," *Quarterly Journal of Economics*, 124(2) pgs 597-636.

[7] Chandra, Amitabh, Jonathan Gruber, and Robin McKnight, (2010), "Patient Cost Sharing and Hospitalization Offsets in the Elderly," *American Economic Review*, 100(1) pgs 193-213.

[8] Cholesterol Treatment Trialists' Collaborators (2005) "Efficacy and safety of cholesterol-lowering treatment: prospective meta-analysis of data from 90,056 participants in 14 randomised trials of statins." *Lancet*. Vol. 366 Pages 1267-1278.

[9] Cholesterol Treatment Trialists' Collaborators (2008) "Efficacy of cholesterol-lowering therapy in 18,686 people with diabetes in 14 randomised trials of statins: a meta-analysis." *Lancet*. Vol. 371 Pages 117-25.

[10] Cholesterol Treatment Trialists' Collaborators (2010) "Efficacy and safety of more intensive lowering of LDL cholesterol: a meta-analysis of data from 170,000 participants in 26 randomised trials" *Lancet*. Vol. 376 Pages 1670-1681.

[11] Cholesterol Treatment Trialists' Collaborators (2012) "The effects of lowering LDL cholesterol with statin therapy in people at low risk of vascular disease: meta-analysis of individual data from 27 randomised trials." *Lancet*. Vol. 380 Pages 581-590.

[12] Congressional Budget Office. 2014. "Competition and the Cost of Medicare's Prescription Drug Program."

[13] Cutler, David, (2004), *Your Money or Your Life: Strong Medicine for America's Healthcare System*, Oxford University Press.

[14] Cutler, David and Wendy Everett, (2010), "Thinking outside the pillbox - medication adherence as a priority for health care reform," *New England Journal of Medicine*, Perspective, 362, pgs 17.

[15] Cutler, David, Genia Long, Ernst Berndt, Jimmy Royer, Andree-Anne Fournier, Alicia Sasser and Pierre Cremieux, (2007), "The Value of Antihypertensive Drugs: A Perspective on Medical Innovation," *Health Affairs*, 26(1) pgs 97-110.

[16] Dahlof, Bjorn, Lars H. Lindholm, Lennart Hansson, Bengt Schersten, Tord Ekbom, P.O. Wester. (1991). "Morbidity and mortality in teh Swedish Trial in Old Patients with Hypertension." *Lancet* Vol. 338. No. 8778.

[17] Deschenes, Olivier and Enrico Moretti. (2009). "Extreme weather events, mortality, and migration." *The Review of Economics and Statistics*. Vol. 91(4). 659-681.

[18] Drukker, David M. (2003) "Testing for serial correlation in linear panel-data models." *The Stata Journal* 3, Number 2, pp. 168-177.

[19] Duggan, Mark and Fiona Scott-Morton, (2010), "The Effect of Medicare Part D on Pharmaceutical Prices and Utilization," American Economic Review, 100(1) pgs 590-607.

[20] Dunn, Abe, (2011), "The Effect of Health Insurance Competition when Private Insurers Compete with a Public Option", BEA Working Paper.

[21] Dunn, Abe, (2012), "Drug Innovations and Welfare Measured Computed from Market Demand: The Case of Anticholesterol Drugs," *American Economic Journal: Applied Economics*, 4(3) pgs 167-89.

[22] Dunn, Abe and Adam Hale Shapiro (2015), "Physician Payments Under Health Care Reform," *Journal of Health Economics*, Vol. 39. pgs. 89-105.

[23] Eaddy, Michael, Christopher Cook, Ken O'Day, Steven Burch, Ron Cantrell, (2012), "How Patient Cost-Sharing Trends Affect Adherence and Outcomes: A Literature Review," *Pharmacy and Therapeutics*, 37(1), pgs 45-55.

[24] Eggleston, Karen, Nilay Shah, Steven Smith, Ernst Berndt, and Joseph Newhouse, (2011), "Quality Adjustment for Health Care Spending on Chronic Disease: Evidence from Diabetes Treatment, 1999-2009," *American Economic Review, Papers and Proceedings*, 101(3), pgs 206-211.

[25] Engelhardt, Gary V., and Jonathan Gruber. 2011. "Medicare Part D and the Financial Protection of the Elderly." *American Economic Journal: Economic Policy*, 3(4): 77-102.

[26] Finkelstein, Amy and Robin McKnight, (2008), "What did Medicare do? The initial impact of Medicare on mortality and out of pocket medical spending," *Journal of Public Economics*, pgs 1644-1668.

[27] Finkelstein, Amy, (2007), "The Aggregate Effects of Health Insurance: Evidence from the Introduction of Medicare," *Quarterly Journal of Economics*, 122(1), pgs 1-37.

[28] Hajat, S., R. Kovats, R. Atkinson, and A. Haines, 2002. "Impact of Hot Temperatures on Death in London: A Time Series Approach,' *Journal of Epidemiology and Community Health* 56 (2002), 367–372.

[29] Khan, Nasreen and Robert Kaestner. 2009. "Effect of Prescription Drug Coverage on the Elderly's Use of Prescription Drugs." *Inquiry*.

[30] Ketcham, Jonathan and Kosali Simon, (2008), "Medicare Part D's Effects on Elderly Drug Costs and Utilization," *American Journal of Managed Care*, November pgs 14-22.

[31] Lakdawalla, Darius and Wesley Yin, (2014), "Insurers' negotiating Leverage and the External Effects of Medicare Part D," *The Review of Economics and Statistics*, forthcoming.

[32] LaRosa, John, Jiang He, and Suma Vupputuri, (1999), "Effects of Statins on Risk of Coronary Disease. A Meta-Analysis of Randomized Controlled Trials," *Journal of the American Medical Association*, 282 pgs 2340-6.

[33] Law, M.R., N.J. Wald, and A.R. Rudnicka, (2003), "Quantifying Effects of Statins on Low Density Lipoprotein Cholesterol, Ischemic Heart Disease, and Stroke: Systematic Review and Meta-Analysis," *BMJ*, 326(28), pgs 1-7.

[34] Lee, R., "Short-Term Variation: Vital Rates, Prices, and Weather", in E. A. Wrigley and R. S. Schofield (Eds.) 1981, *The Population History of England 1541–1871*

[35] Levy, Helen, Meltzer, David, 2004. "What do we really know about whether health insurance affects health?" In: McLaughlin, Catherine (Ed.), Health Policy on the Uninsured: Setting the Agenda. Urban Institute Press.

[36] Lichtenberg, Frank R. and Shawn X. Sun. 2007. "The Impact of Medicare Part D on Prescription Drug Use by the Elderly." *Health Affairs*.

[37] Newhouse, J. P. and the Insurance Experiment Group (1993). "Free for all? Lessons from the RAND Health Insurance Experiment," Cambridge, MA: Harvard University Press.

[38] Nickell, Stephen, (1981), "Biases in Dynamic Models with Fixed Effects," *Econometrica*, 49, pgs 1417-26.

[39] Ruhm, Christopher, (2000), "Are recessions good for your health?" *Quarterly Journal of Economics*, 115(2) pgs 618-650.

[40] Schwartz, Joel. (2001), "Is there harvesting in the association of airborne particles with daily deaths and hospital admissions?" *Epidemiology*. Vol 12(1). pgs.55-61.

[41] SHEP Cooperative Research Group, (1991), "Prevention of stroke by antihypertensive drug treatment in older persons with isolated systolic hypertension." *Journal of the American Medical Association*, 265(24) pgs 3255-3264.

[42] Solomon, Matthew, Dana Goldman, Geoffrey Joyce, Jose Escarce, (2009), "Cost-sharing and the initiation of drug therapy for the chronically ill," *Archive of Internal Medicine*, 169(8).

[43] Veterans Administration Cooperative Study Group on Antihypertension Agents, (1967), "Effects of Morbidity on Treatment for Hypertension: Results in Patients with Diastolic Blood Pressures Averaging 115 Through 129 mm Hg," *Journal of the American Medical Association*,

[44] Veterans Administration Cooperative Study Group on Antihypertension Agents, (1970), "Effects of Morbidity on Treatment for Hypertension II. Results in Patients with Diastolic Blood Pressure Average 90 Through 114 mm Hg," *Journal of the American Medical Association,*

Appendix

A Demand Analysis

We estimate equation (7) with the out-of-pocket expenditure share as an endogenous covariate and the expected impact of Part D as an instrumental variable for the out-of-pocket share. Specifically, we estimate the following equation:

$$E_{i,t,c} = \exp(\alpha_c + \gamma_t + \phi_d \log(\frac{oopc_{i,t,c}}{E_{i,t,c}}) + \beta Z_{i,t,c} + \zeta_{i,t,c}) + v_{i,t,c}. \qquad (9)$$

However, the generosity of the insurance, as captured by $\log(\frac{oopc_{i,t,c}}{E_{i,t,c}})$, is endogenous in this specification, since those with the greatest health problems will purchase more insurance. Specifically, there may be a correlation between $\log(\frac{oopc_{i,t,c}}{E_{i,t,c}})$ and the unobserved factors expressed by the error term $\zeta_{i,t,c}$. To address this endogeneity problem we use $\Delta INS_c \cdot Post_t$ as an instrument in a two-stage residual inclusion model. Specifically, we estimate equation (8) in a first stage in order to provide a consistent estimate of unobserved factors that may be related to out-of-pocket expenditure share, $\widehat{\zeta}_{i,t,c} = \log(\frac{oopc_{i,t,c}}{E_{i,t,c}}) - \widehat{\alpha}_c + \widehat{\gamma}_t + \widehat{\tau}_d \Delta INS_c \cdot Post_t + \widehat{\beta} Z_{i,t,c}$. Including $\widehat{\zeta}_{i,t,c}$ in (9) controls for the unobserved factors that could bias the estimate of ϕ_d. This offers an alternative and more direct estimate of consumer demand that can be directly compared with well-known studies in the literature.[60]

The estimates of the demand model are included in Table A1. Model 1 shows the GLM estimates without instrumenting. The estimates show a highly significant and negative relationship between expenditures and the out-of-pocket share, which is likely biased downward because of selection. The following Models 2-4 estimate the model using the residual inclusion approach, but applying distinct functional forms. Model 2 excludes the health information of the individual while Models 3 and 4 include this information. The GLM Model 4 uses a Gamma distributional assumption, rather than a Poisson, but the estimated elasticity changes very little. The absolute value of the elasticities is significantly smaller than in Model 1, highlighting the importance of applying instrumental variable estimates.

---

[60]Although expenditure is a left-hand side variable, it should be noted that the demand estimation is likely capturing a quantity effect, since the county and time fixed effects likely account for any drug price differences across markets and over time. In addition, the out-of-pocket share variable, $\frac{oopc_{i,t,c}}{E_{i,t,c}}$, and many changes in price may not impact this ratio. For example, if a policy covers 80 percent of expenditures, a price change does not affect this ratio.

Table A1: Predicted Change in Drug Insurance on Total and Out-of-Pocket Drug Expenditures

	(1)	(2)	(3)	(4)
log(out-of-pocket share)	-0.360***	-0.176	-0.195*	-0.262**
	(0.010)	(0.113)	(0.115)	(0.123)
Residual Inclusion		-0.185	-0.125	-0.143
		(0.114)	(0.115)	(0.124)
Log(BMI)	0.667***	0.733***	0.347***	0.445***
	(0.044)	(0.053)	(0.046)	(0.049)
Log(Income)	0.082***	0.059***	0.099***	0.075***
	(0.012)	(0.018)	(0.018)	(0.016)
Arteriosclerotic H.D.			0.195***	0.246***
			(0.022)	(0.025)
Hypertension			0.218***	0.317***
			(0.020)	(0.020)
Heart Attack			0.028	0.037
			(0.040)	(0.050)
Angina/CHD			0.119***	0.162***
			(0.032)	(0.033)
Other Heart Problems			0.063**	0.091***
			(0.030)	(0.029)
Diabetes			0.281***	0.341***
			(0.020)	(0.022)
Observations	30451	30451	30448	30448
Instrument	No	Yes	Yes	Yes
Model	GLM, Poisson	GLM, Poisson	GLM, Poisson	GLM, Gamma

Notes: All regressions include county and year fixed effects, as well as controls for demographics (i.e. age, sex, race, education). Standard errors clustered by county. $^*p < 0.10$, $^{**}p < 0.05$, $^{***}p < 0.01$.

B   Predicted Effects of Part D: Medicare HMO and Medicaid Penetration Rates

Two determinants of drug coverage before the reform are the availability of drug insurance through Medicaid or the Medicare Advantage program. Both of these programs are influenced by external factors. Recall that Medicaid will be affected by different eligibility requirements across states and Medicare Advantage penetration is also affected by a multitude of fairly exogenous factors (e.g., regulatory rates set by CMS, private commercial insurers in the area, and sufficient population for economies of scale for an HMO).

As a robustness exercise, we use the penetration rates of these two programs before Part D reform as instrumental variables for the change in drug coverage at the before the reform. This instrumental variable approach aims to evaluate the effects on coverage that are related to these two known differences in prescription drug coverage across markets prior to the reform. A key reason for applying these values as instruments is to correct for potential measurement error in the insurance change variable. The first stage of the instrumental variable estimation is:

$$\Delta INS_c \cdot Post_t = \beta_1 MCAID_s^{2005} \cdot Post_t + \beta_2 HMO_c^{2005} \cdot Post_t + \beta_d X_{d,t,c} + \gamma_{d,c} + \gamma_{d,t} + \xi_{d,t,c},$$

where $MCAID_s^{2005}$ represents the Medicaid state penetration in 2005 and HMO_c^{2005} represents the Medicare Advantage penetration in the county in 2005.[61] As expected, those areas with higher rates of Medicaid and Medicare Advantage penetration are significantly less impacted by the reform. The relationship between these key variables is reported in Table B1. In addition to our main sample used in the text, we also estimate an alternative model that includes less populated counties. This is done for additional identification power, since Medicare Advantage HMO plans tend not to enter more rural areas.

Table B1: Relationship Between Change in Insurance and Pre-reform Medicaid Share and Pre-reform Medicare Advantage Penetration

	(1)	(2)
Share Medicaid in 2005	-0.246	-0.228
	(0.169)	(0.162)
Unemployment Rate in 2005	-0.042	-0.037
	(0.071)	(0.070)
Medicare Advantage Penetration in 2005	-0.262***	-0.278***
	(0.062)	(0.061)
Observations	169	179
Min. 65+ Cty. Pop	2,000	None

Notes: Estimate is based on 2006 data only. The model includes other covariates in the mortality regression, including age distribution and unemployment. The actual IV estimate is based on these relationships, but including interactions for treatment and post-reform fixed effects. "Min. 65+ Cty. Pop." indicates the 65+ population of the smallest county used in the sample, taken from the 2000 Census. $*p < 0.10$, $**p < 0.05$, $***p < 0.01$.

The instrumental variable estimates are reported in Table B2.[62] The qualitative results do not change from the results in the paper, although the magnitude of the effect of

---

[61]We also include an interaction of the unemployment rate in 2005 with the post variable, since the number of individuals on Medicaid is influenced by the local economic environment.

[62]For the Medicaid variable, we also include an interaction of the Medicaid eligibility prior to the reform with the unemployment rate in 2005, since the number of individuals on Medicaid is influenced by the local

receiving drug insurance on mortality is substantially greater.

Table B2: Logit Competing-Risks Model - Medicaid and Medicare Advantage IVs

	(1)	(2)	(3)	(4)
Change*Post*Cardio	-0.306	-0.309*	-0.514**	-0.492**
	(0.190)	(0.178)	(0.211)	(0.198)
Change*Post*NonCardio	-0.070	-0.066	0.117	0.091
	(0.117)	(0.116)	(0.149)	(0.153)
Observations	2028	2028	2148	2148
Mortality Measure	Years-of-life Lost	Mortality	Years-of-life Lost	Mortality
Min. 65+ Cty. Pop	2,000	2,000	None	None

Notes: The mortality share measures used in the above estimates are based the age 65 to 84 population. All regressions include county-disease fixed effects, year-disease fixed effects, the age distribution of the population and the unemployment rate. "Min. 65+ Cty. Pop." indicates the 65+ population of the smallest county used in the sample, taken from the 2000 Census. Standard errors clustered by county. $^*p < 0.10$, $^{**}p < 0.05$, $^{***}p < 0.01$.

C   Nested Logit

To estimate a nested logit model, we add a third type of mortality category that includes individuals who die of a noncardiovascular illness, and are recorded as having a cardiovascular comorbidity at the time of their death. This third mortality category draws upon additional medical condition information from the CDC mortality data, which lists all of an individual's major conditions at the time of death. Thus, the three different causes of death considered in the analysis are cardiovascular death, noncardiovascular death with cardiovascular comorbidity, and noncardiovascular death without cardiovascular comorbidity. The share of individuals dying in each of these categories is 40 percent, 23 percent, and 37 percent, respectively. Column (1) of Table C1 presents the results of the estimates with the three mortality categories included. The estimates show a significant decline in cardiovascular-related mortality, as in the previous results. However, we see an increase in noncardiovascular-related deaths with a cardiovascular comorbidity, although

---

economic environment. As expected, those areas with higher rates of Medicaid and Medicare Advantage penetration are significantly less impacted by the reform. The first-stage estimates show the instruments to be strong and the Sargan test of overidentifying restrictions cannot reject the null hypothesis that the instruments are uncorrelated with the error term.

this estimate is not statistically significant. However, the positive sign is consistent with individuals surviving their cardiovascular illness, but dying of other causes.

The nested logit model follows from the fact that the error term, $\epsilon_{d,t,c,i}$, then has two components, including an i.i.d. shock and another group-specific component. In our analysis we select a nesting structure that includes those who die of a cardiovascular illness and those who die of a noncardiovascular illness with a cardiovascular comorbidity within the same nest. That is, one can think of the group-specific shock as capturing the prevalence of cardiovascular comorbidities in the population. Berry (1994) shows that this type of nesting structure may be incorporated into linear estimation of equation (4) by adding the nesting term, $\log\left(\frac{s_d}{s_{cardio}+s_{noncardio\ w/\ cardio\ comorbidity}}\right)$.

Table C1: Nested Logit Model

	(1)	(2)	(3)	(4)
Change*Cardio*Post	-0.229***	-0.309***	-0.221***	-0.222***
	(0.082)	(0.093)	(0.068)	(0.068)
Change*NonCardio w/CardioComorb*Post	0.082	0.075	-0.056	
	(0.102)	(0.105)	(0.072)	
Change*NonCardio w/o CardioComorb*Post	0.016	0.083	0.105	
	(0.078)	(0.084)	(0.086)	
Cardio*$\delta_{cardio,0}$		0.657***	0.459***	0.460***
		(0.086)	(0.093)	(0.093)
NonCardio w/ CardioComorb*$\delta_{cardio,0}$		0.807***	0.487***	0.489***
		(0.064)	(0.062)	(0.062)
NonCardio w/o CardioComorb*$\delta_{cardio,0}$		0.913***	0.935***	0.935***
		(0.047)	(0.048)	(0.048)
Nesting Parameter			0.573***	0.571***
			(0.069)	(0.069)
Observations	3006	2505	2505	2505
Sample Years	2000-04, 2006	2001-04, 2006	2001-04, 2006	2001-04, 2006
County-Disease FE	Yes	No	No	No
County FE	No	Yes	Yes	Yes
Instrumental Variables	No	Yes	Yes	Yes

Notes: The share measures used in the above estimates are based on the years-of-life lost for the 65 to 84 population. All regressions include county-disease fixed effects, year-disease fixed effects, the age distribution of the population and the unemployment rate. Standard errors clustered by county. $^*p < 0.10$, $^{**}p < 0.05$, $^{***}p < 0.01$.

The inclusion of this additional term creates two complications. First, the term is endogenous, since the share term is contained within the dependent variable, so we will need to estimate the model using instrumental variables. Second, the inclusion of disease-county fixed effects removes much of the variation from the model, which complicates trying to find appropriate instruments for the nesting term. To address these issues we first specify a model similar to column (1) that allows for more degrees of freedom. Rather than including disease-county fixed effects, the estimate in column (2) includes only county fixed effects along with disease fixed effects that are common across counties. To capture county-specific health, the estimate in column (2) includes the value of the dependent variable in 2000 as an additional covariate.[63] Although many more degrees of freedom are added by the exclusion of the disease-specific fixed effects, the estimate in column (2) is quite similar to those of column (1). A likely reason for this is that mortality rates by disease are specific to each county and persistent, so the mortality in 2000 is a strong predictor of mortality in future periods.

With the additional nesting term included, the nested logit regression model becomes:

$$\delta_{d,t,c} = \delta_{0,t,c} + \tau_d \cdot \Delta\widehat{INS}_c \cdot Post_t \tag{10}$$
$$+ \ \beta X_{d,t,c} + \sigma \ln\left(\frac{s_{d\in\{cardio, noncardio \ w/ \ cardio \ comorb.\}}}{s_{cardio} + s_{noncardio \ w/ \ cardio \ comorb.}}\right)$$
$$+ \ \gamma_c + \gamma_{d,t} + \xi_{d,t,c} \tag{11}$$

where $\delta_{0,t,c}$ is the value of the dependent variable in 2000. With the additional degrees of freedom, we then choose two specific instruments to address the endogeneity concerns. One instrument is the value of the nesting term for the population that is 55-64 years old. The nesting term of this younger population within the same county may be correlated through common health factors affecting the entire population, but should also be exogenous, since the population is distinct and should be less directly affected by Part D than those over 65. The two-period lag value of the nesting term is also used as an instrument for the current period nest. The two-period lag is used since it covers the mortality rate of the same disease category within the same county and the instrument is derived from data prior to the Part D implementation.[64]

The results of the nested logit model are reported in column (3). The nesting parameter is shown to be large and statistically significant, implying strong substitution between

---

[63]Since the mortality in 2000 is added to the specification, we limit the pre-period sample to 2002-04. We could include 2001 in the Model 2 specification with similar results. However, for the model that includes a nest, Model 3, we use the two-period lag of the nesting term as an instrument, implying 2001 must be dropped from Model 3. To keep the estimates comparable, 2001 is also dropped from Model 2.

[64]We use a two-period lag, rather than a one-period lag, so that the transition period, 2005, is not included as an instrument. This assumption is not critical: using a single lag, rather than a two-period lag, produces qualitatively similar results.

cardiovascular-related deaths and noncardiovascular-related deaths where a cardiovascular comorbidity is present, as might be expected. Similar to the previous estimates, column (3) also shows a significant reduction in cardiovascular-related deaths. However, distinct from columns (1) and (2) we see no increase in noncardiovascular death with a cardiovascular comorbidity. That is, it appears that the increase in this type of mortality, reflected in columns (1) and (2), may be caused by substitution patterns that were not accounted for in previous models. The effects on cardiovascular-related mortality is negative and significant in column (3), but less precisely estimated than prior estimates.

Overall, the estimates reported in Table C highlight that our results are robust to alternative specifications of the logit framework. However, there are several alternatives to the nested logic framework that are computationally more intensive, but allow for greater flexibility in specifying the alternative substitution patterns that may lead to new insights. This appears to be a useful area for future research.

D   Additional Tables

Table D1: Cause of Death by ICD-9 Disease Chapter for 65 and Over Population

Cause of Death Chapter	Share of Deaths
hline Diseases of the circulatory system	40.4%
Neoplasms	21.1%
Diseases of the respiratory system	11.3%
Mental Illness	7.8%
Endocrine; nutritional; and metabolism	4.0%
Diseases of the genitourinary system	2.8%
Diseases of the digestive system	2.7%
Diseases of the nervous system	1.9%
Infectious and parasitic diseases	1.8%
Other	6.1%

Table D2: Demographic Differences in Drug Coverage

Age-Sex Category	Pre-Part D (2004-05)	Post Part D (2006-07)	Change		Avg. Annual Pop. (Thousands)
Male					
65-69	68.3%	84.1%	15.8%	16,089	4,022
70-74	69.1%	86.2%	17.1%	13,892	3,473
75-79	68.8%	87.5%	18.6%	12,502	3,125
80-84	66.3%	87.0%	20.8%	8,708	2,177
85+	61.0%	84.3%	23.2%	6,167	1,542
Female					
65-69	73.4%	86.8%	13.4%	18,660	4,665
70-74	73.6%	91.0%	17.4%	17,308	4,327
75-79	70.0%	89.7%	19.7%	15,193	3,798
80-84	67.2%	88.3%	21.1%	13,303	3,326
85+	54.6%	86.2%	31.5%	14,094	3,523
s.d. by age-sex category	5.7%	2.2%	5.0%		
s.d. by age-sex category (Under 85)	2.7%	2.1%	2.6%		

Table D3: Probit: Predicted Drug Coverage by County

	Pre Reform	Post Reform
Age 65 to 69	0.513***	0.172*
	(0.075)	(0.093)
Age 70 to 74	0.497***	0.185**
	(0.075)	(0.093)
Age 75 to 79	0.463***	0.290***
	(0.075)	(0.094)
Age 80 to 84	0.351***	0.237**
	(0.076)	(0.094)
Age 85 to 90	0.285***	0.138
	(0.082)	(0.101)
Male*(Age 65 to 69)	0.118***	0.159***
	(0.045)	(0.055)
Male*(Age 70 to 74)	0.130***	0.314***
	(0.045)	(0.057)
Male*(Age 75 to 79)	0.008	0.117**
	(0.045)	(0.059)
Male*(Age 80 to 84)	0.038	0.104*
	(0.045)	(0.056)
Male*(Age 85 to 89)	-0.126**	0.153**
	(0.057)	(0.069)
Male*(Age 90+)	-0.231***	0.103
	(0.077)	(0.097)
Observations	18651	18409

Table D4: Independent-Risks Model: Robustness to Alternative Mortality Measures

	Overall			Cardiovascular			Noncardiovascular		
Age 65 to 84, Age-Sex Adjusted Years-of-life Lost									
Change*Post	-0.061***	-0.041**	-0.065**	-0.037***	-0.040***	-0.050***	-0.023	-0.001	-0.016
	(0.021)	(0.018)	(0.032)	(0.012)	(0.011)	(0.018)	(0.017)	(0.015)	(0.024)
Age 65+, Age-Sex Adjusted Years-of-life Lost									
Change*Post	-0.046**	-0.040**	-0.059*	-0.025**	-0.034***	-0.045**	-0.021	-0.006	-0.013
	(0.023)	(0.019)	(0.033)	(0.012)	(0.010)	(0.021)	(0.017)	(0.015)	(0.022)
Age 65 to 84, Age-Sex Adjusted Mortality Rate									
Change*Post	-0.005***	-0.003*	-0.005*	-0.003***	-0.003***	-0.004***	-0.002	0.000	0.000
	(0.002)	(0.002)	(0.003)	(0.001)	(0.001)	(0.002)	(0.002)	(0.001)	(0.001)
Age 65+, Age-Sex Adjusted Mortality Rate									
Change*Post	-0.003	-0.003	-0.005	-0.002	-0.003**	-0.004	-0.001	-0.000	-0.001
	(0.003)	(0.002)	(0.004)	(0.001)	(0.001)	(0.002)	(0.002)	(0.002)	(0.002)
Observations	507	1014	1014	507	1014	1014	507	1014	1014
Sample Years	2003-04, 2006	2000-04, 2006	2000-04, 2006	2003-04, 2006	2000-04, 2006	2000-04, 2006	2003-04, 2006	2000-04, 2006	2000-04, 2006
County Specific Trend	No	No	Yes	No	No	Yes	No	No	Yes

Notes: Overall mortality includes individuals who died from any cause. Cardiovascular mortality includes only individuals who died from a cardiovascular related disease as the primary cause of death. noncardiovascular mortality includes only individuals who died from a noncardiovascular related-disease as the primary cause of death. *Post* indicates a post-reform dummy. All regressions include county fixed effects, year dummies, the age distribution of the population, and the unemployment rate. Standard errors clustered by county. $* p < 0.10$, $** p < 0.05$, $*** p < 0.01$.

Table D5: Counties Used in Main Analysis

State	County	State	County	State	County
Alabama	Butler	Michigan	Cheboygan	Oklahoma	Comanche
	Colbert		Emmet	Pennsylvania	Allegheny
	Jefferson		Genesee		Bucks
	Lauderdale		Hillsdale		Cambria
	Madison		Kent		Chester
Arizona	Maricopa		Macomb		Delaware
	Pima		Muskegon		Lackawanna
Arkansas	Benton		Oakland		Lehigh
	Washington		Presque Isle		Luzerne
California	Contra Costa		Roscommon		Montgomery
	Los Angeles		Wayne		Northampton
	Orange	Minnesota	Benton		Philadelphia
	Riverside		Dakota		Potter
	Sacramento		Hennepin		Somerset
	San Bernardino		Stearns	South Carolina	Darlington
	San Diego	Missouri	Dunklin		Marlboro
	San Francisco		Pulaski	Tennessee	Cumberland
	San Joaquin		St. Charles		Decatur
	San Mateo		St. Louis		Hamilton
Colorado	Denver	Nebraska	Dawson		Hardin
	Jefferson	Nevada	Clark		Wayne
Connecticut	Hartford		Elko		White
	Middlesex	New Jersey	Bergen	Texas	Dallas
Florida	Broward		Camden		Gillespie
	DeSoto		Middlesex		Gregg
	Flagler		Ocean		Harris
	Hillsborough		Passaic		Harrison
	Lee		Union		Hays
	Manatee	New Mexico	Santa Fe		Kerr
	Palm Beach	New York	Bronx		Montgomery
	Pasco		Broome		Polk
	Pinellas		Clinton		Tarrant
	Polk		Kings		Travis
	Volusia		Monroe		Tyler
Georgia	Colquitt		Nassau		Williamson
	Fulton		New York	Virginia	Chesterfield
	Walker		Onondaga		Fairfax
	Whitfield		Oswego		Henrico
	Worth		Queens		Richmond City
Illinois	Cook		Suffolk	Washington	King
	DuPage		Westchester		Kitsap
	Kane	North Carolina	Cleveland		Mason
	Saline		Forsyth		Pierce
	Will		Guilford	West Virginia	Braxton
Iowa	Lee		Mecklenburg		Hancock
Kansas	Johnson		Pitt		Nicholas
	Shawnee		Randolph	Wisconsin	Brown
Kentucky	Jefferson		Robeson		Dane
	Union		Rowan		Milwaukee
Louisiana	East Baton Rouge		Scotland		Waukesha
Maryland	Anne Arundel	Ohio	Clinton	Wyoming	Sweetwater
	Baltimore		Cuyahoga		
	Montgomery		Fairfield		
	Prince George's		Franklin		
Massachusetts	Essex		Hamilton		
	Middlesex		Jefferson		
	Norfolk		Lorain		
	Plymouth		Ottawa		
	Suffolk		Williams		

Notes: These are the 169 counties used for the main analysis in the study. These counties have age 65+ populations greater than 2,000 (in the year 2000) and have at least 30 sample points available over the 2004 to 2005 time period in the MCBS.

Table D6: Logit Competing-Risks Model: Mortality Shares as Dependent Variable

	(1)	(2)	(3)	(4)
Change*Post*Cardio	-0.190***	-0.193**	-0.274***	-0.271**
	(0.073)	(0.075)	(0.080)	(0.109)
Change*Post*NonCardio	-0.052	0.036	-0.045	-0.047
	(0.067)	(0.060)	(0.097)	(0.089)
Observations	1014	2028	2028	2028
Sample Years	2003-04, 2006	2000-04, 2006	2000-04, 2006	2000-04, 2006
County-Disease FE	Yes	Yes	Yes	Yes
County Specific Trend	No	No	Yes	No
County-Disease Specific Trend	No	No	No	Yes

Notes: The mortality share measures used in the above estimates are the simple mortality shares for age 65 to 84 population. All regressions include county-disease fixed effects, year-disease fixed effects, the age distribution of the population, and the unemployment rate. Standard errors clustered by county. $^{*}p < 0.10$, $^{**}p < 0.05$, $^{***}p < 0.01$.

Table D7: Logit Competing-Risks Model: Robustness to Alternative Construction of County-Specific Change in Insurance Coverage

	(1)	(2)	(3)	(4)	(5)
Change*Cardio*Post	-0.223***	-0.191***	-0.239***	-0.141**	-0.232**
	(0.083)	(0.069)	(0.073)	(0.071)	(0.113)
Change*NonCardio*Post	0.019	0.032	0.029	0.022	0.032
	(0.056)	(0.054)	(0.055)	(0.043)	(0.069)
Observations	2028	2028	2028	2028	8016
Min MCBS Cty. Sample	30	30	30	30	30
Probit Used to Construct Shares	Yes	No	Yes	Yes	Yes
MCBS Pre Years	2004-2005	2004-2005	2004-2005	2000-2003	2004-2005
MCBS Post Years	2006-2007	2006-2007	2006-2007	2007-2008	2006-2007
Age-Sex Specific Coverage Change	No	No	No	No	Yes
Probit Control Variables	Age, Sex	None	Age, Sex, Health, Educ., Race	Age, Sex	Age, Sex

Notes: The mortality measure used in the above estimates is based on the years-of-life lost for the 65 to 84 population. Sample years are 2001, 2002, 2003, 2004, 2006. All regressions include county-disease fixed effects, year-disease fixed effects, and the age distribution of the population and the unemployment rate. 'Min MCSB Cty. Sample" indicates the MCBS county sample size threshold for dropping counties. "MCBS Pre Years" indicates the years used to calculate $SHARE_c^{pre}$. "MCBS Post Years" indicates the years used to calculate $SHARE_c^{post}$. "Probit used to construct shares" indicates whether a probit model or simple raw counts of the MCBS data were used to calculate $SHARE_c^{pre}$ and $SHARE_c^{post}$. "Probit control variables" indicate the covariates included in the probit regression used to calculate $SHARE_c^{pre}$ and $SHARE_c^{post}$. "Health" indicates comorbidity dummy variables based on disease categories from MCBS. See Section 6.2.3 for a description of how the "Age-Sex specific coverage change" was created. Standard errors clustered by county. *$p < 0.10$, **$p < 0.05$, ***$p < 0.01$.

www.ingramcontent.com/pod-product-compliance
Lightning Source LLC
Chambersburg PA
CBHW081246280526
45787CB00006B/2817